# The Woman's Heart

## AN OWNER'S GUIDE

JOHN A. ELEFTERIADES, MD
and TERESA CAULIN-GLASER, MD

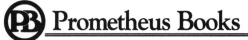 **Prometheus Books**
59 John Glenn Drive
Amherst, New York 14228-2119

Published 2008 by Prometheus Books

Inquiries should be addressed to
Prometheus Books
59 John Glenn Drive
Amherst, New York 14228–2119
VOICE: 716–691–0133, ext. 210
FAX: 716–691–0317
WWW.PROMETHEUSBOOKS.COM

12 11 10 09 08    5 4 3 2 1

Library of Congress Cataloging-in-Publication Data

Elefteriades, John A.
    The woman's heart : an owner's guide / John A. Elefteriades, Teresa Caulin-Glaser.—1st American pbk. ed.
        p. cm.
    Includes bibliographical references and index.
    ISBN 978–1–59102–562–7
    1. Heart diseases in women—Popular works. I Caulin-Glaser, Teresa. II Title.

RC672.E44 2008
616.1'20082—dc22

2007050589

Printed in the United States on acid-free paper

# CONTENTS

# ACKNOWLEDGMENT

The authors would like to thank Alex Baker of DNA Illustrations for her superb artwork in this book.

# PREFACE

*Vive la difference*, so the saying goes, emphasizing the wondrous dissimilarities between men and women. These differences make the world go 'round; without them, the world would be boring and biologically unsustainable. How marvelously intriguing and complicated the world has been thanks to the fascinating interplay of the sexes since earliest civilization. In the past several decades, efforts to achieve equality between the sexes have made great inroads to balance the representation of women in education, employment, and politics. But are we failing to appreciate the important differences?

When it comes to the health of hearts, the differences between men and women can have serious consequences. Because heart disease in women is often dissimilar to that of men, our medical system has been guilty of underrecognition and substandard scientific investigation and clinical treatment of women's heart disease.

The quintessential image of angina (the medical term for chest pain or discomfort due to disease of the blood vessels of the heart) usually shows a middle-aged man clutching his chest in agony. See the adjoining figure.

This is the mental picture imprinted in physicians' consciousness from the first day of medical school. The physician has not been conditioned to think immediately of coronary heart disease in the female patient. Women, we are beginning to realize, may not feel heart attack pain in the same way men do. By virtue of her hormonal protections, the woman was considered to be practically immune to coronary artery disease until well after the change of life. This assumption likely affects how physicians regard the threat of a heart attack in their female patients. It also often prevents

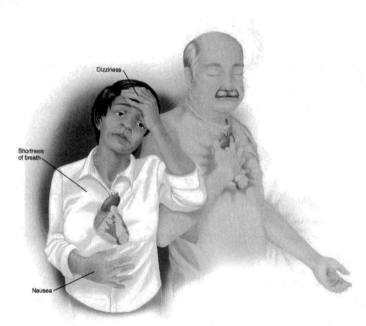

The way a woman feels angina. Note the marked difference from the way a man feels heart pain.

women from being appropriately screened for risk factors for heart disease before they reach menopause or have a heart attack.

For decades, virtually no scientific research addressed the specific manifestations of heart diseases in women. This phenomenon led to powerful regulations from the National Institutes of Health requiring enhanced enrollment of female subjects in heart research. In recent years, study after study has shown that heart disease eludes detection in women, even in the hands of otherwise superbly trained and widely experienced physicians. Furthermore, once heart disease is diagnosed, aggressive treatment and secondary preventive therapies in women are often less optimal as compared with those for men.

The concept that women are immune to heart disease is, simply put, a fallacy. After menopause, women catch up very quickly to men in the prevalence of coronary artery disease. Equally important, in women younger than fifty who do suffer a heart attack, the statistics are frightening: these women are twice as likely to die during their hospitalization for the heart attack as compared with men.

Consider the following sobering facts:

## INCIDENCE OF HEART DISEASE IN WOMEN

MYTH:   Breast cancer is the number-one killer of women.

FACT:    Cardiovascular disease kills the most women. While breast cancer claims 42,000 women in the United States each year, cardiovascular disease accounts for the deaths of 500,000 women in the United States annually. In fact, three times as many women die of heart disease each year as from all cancers combined. Virtually half of all female deaths are caused by heart disease.

MYTH:   Only men are affected by heart attacks.

FACT:    More women than men die of heart attacks each year. This has been true since 1984. Currently, women represent nearly 55 percent of all deaths from cardiovascular disease.

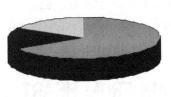 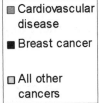

Contributions of cancer and heart disease to death of women.

## SYMPTOMS OF HEART DISEASE IN WOMEN

MYTH:   Women and men have the same symptoms during a heart attack.

FACT:    Women are often delayed in seeking or receiving care for heart attacks.

The symptoms of heart attack may be different in women than in men. Men more often experience the classic chest pain and pressure, while in women, the symptoms may manifest themselves only as gastrointestinal discomfort/pain, shortness of breath, shoulder/arm/upper-back discomfort/pain, nausea, jaw pain, extreme fatigue, dizziness, or any combination of these.

The woman herself or the treating physician may fail to recognize the symptoms and to reach the correct diagnosis.

## RISKS OF TREATMENTS FOR CORONARY ARTERY DISEASE

MYTH:   Women and men have the same outcomes with surgery and angioplasty.

FACT:   Since the inception of open-heart surgery some thirty-five years ago, the mortality rate for women undergoing coronary artery bypass grafting has been higher than that for men by about twofold. The same holds true for angioplasty. Both phenomena are thought to be due to the smaller size of women's coronary arteries, which predisposes them to graft- or angioplasty-site closure.

## NATURAL PROTECTION FROM HEART DISEASE UNTIL MENOPAUSE

MYTH:   Only postmenopausal women are at risk for heart disease or have heart attacks.

FACT:   Generally, women are protected from coronary artery disease until menopause. However, this is not absolute. Before the change of life, vascular disease is held in check by the woman's hormones as well as a low likelihood of cardiac risk factors. The occurrence of heart disease in younger women is usually related to the presence of very strong risk factors such as a family history of heart disease, tobacco use, diabetes mellitus, or markedly abnormal cholesterol levels. Unfortunately, with the increasing incidence of obesity, smoking, inactivity, hypertension, and diabetes in teenagers and young women, we may see heart disease at increasingly younger ages in the future.

## A TENDENCY FOR CERTAIN HEART DISEASES AMONG WOMEN

MYTH:   Men are at higher risk for all types of heart problems, compared with women.

FACT:   Although we tend to think of heart disease as a male phenomenon, certain cardiac illnesses actually occur more commonly in women. Among those cardiac diseases are mitral valve prolapse, rheumatic fever, and ulcers of the aorta (the main artery of the body).

## DIFFICULTY OF DIAGNOSTIC TESTING IN WOMEN

MYTH:   The accuracy of diagnostic testing for heart disease is equal in men and women.

FACT:   Some noninvasive testing for heart disease can often lead to false positive results in women (that is, the test result suggests that heart disease is present when it is not). For example, in one of the most useful diagnostic tests for coronary artery disease—the nuclear stress test—the images can be misleading for one simple reason: the shadow of the left breast obscures the camera's view of the heart's shadow.

# SEVERITY OF HEART DISEASE IN WOMEN

MYTH:   Women are more likely to have "mild" heart disease.

FACT:   Women find themselves at much more advanced stages of heart muscle damage by the time the heart disease is diagnosed than do men.

MYTH:   Men are more likely than woman to die from a heart attack.

FACT:   Heart attacks are more lethal in women than in men up to the age of seventy-five, when the death rates become equal. Younger women have a particularly high risk for death from a heart attack, compared with younger men.

MYTH:   A woman who has not had a heart attack is not at risk for developing heart failure.

FACT:   Almost 63 percent of deaths from heart failure occur in women. Untreated high blood pressure places a woman at a greater risk to develop heart failure compared with a man—even if she has never had a heart attack.

For all these reasons, it is imperative that women be well informed about recognition and treatment of heart illness.

This book is dedicated to the woman's heart. We examine the differences in the structure and function of the heart in women, exploring the effects of hormonal influence as well as the phases of the lifecycle. We provide a description of the symptoms of heart disease specific to women. We visit fully the issue of hormone therapy after menopause. We explain differences in treatment patterns and results of treatment in women.

We will address the following specific topics and questions:

- How does my heart work?
- What changes occur to my heart and circulation during pregnancy and delivery?
- How is my heart different from a man's?
- How can I recognize a heart attack?
- Does being overweight increase my risk of heart disease?
- Is hormone therapy a good idea for me?
- Is mitral valve prolapse really a serious condition?
- How can I prevent heart disease?
- How do women fare with heart therapies?
- What happens to my heart as I age?
- Will I pass on heart disease to my children and grandchildren as a genetic legacy?
- What prospects promise to improve heart health and treatment?
- How can I cope, emotionally and physically, with the burden of knowing I have heart disease?

(You may notice some overlap of information about specific topics among different chapters. This is intentional so that you will have as many facts as possible readily available when reading a chapter.)

Our goal is, quite simply, to provide you with an "owner's manual" for your female heart. We want you to be more attuned to symptoms of heart disease. If you should develop or currently suffer from heart disease, we aim to make you well versed on general options and expectations.

We hope that you will enjoy and learn from the information in the pages that follow as much as we did in compiling and preparing it.

We want to teach you to live with your heart in a healthy way and, we hope, to live a fruitful life for a very long time.

# INTRODUCTION: THE "BROKEN HEART" SYNDROME

There is no more dramatic way to demonstrate just how different the woman's heart is than by acquainting you with the broken heart syndrome.

Maureen was fifty-five. She had just made it through menopause. She had been married for thirty-two years to a pharmaceutical executive. Their three daughters were happily married and living in different parts of the world. Maureen herself had an important administrative position at a major Midwestern health clinic. She and her husband had had some differences over the years, but the duration of their experience and their common love of their children would always keep them together—or so she thought. She drove to her suburban home one night after work to find the doors barred, the locks changed, and an envelope taped to the front door. The letter from her husband indicated he had left her for his high school sweetheart and gone to the Bahamas. She should find another place to live, he said. She wept on the doorstep for about an hour before driving to her best friend's house. Her comfortable life had, in an instant, been rent asunder. She was on the highway when the pains came on. Her chest hurt so badly that she swerved toward oncoming traffic. She was barely able to regain control and bring the car to rest on the grassy median.

The next thing Maureen remembered was being

wheeled into the cardiac catheterization suite. She could grasp only bits and pieces of what the doctors and nurses were telling her. She was having a heart attack, they said. Her echocardiogram (echo) showed abnormalities. Her EKG indicated more than half her heart was not functioning. She had to have an urgent catheterization to find which artery was closed and to open it immediately.

As it turned out, her arteries were *clean*. She had *no* arteriosclerosis. She was merely suffering from a "broken heart."

She was, however, in cardiogenic shock, a serious, advanced state of heart failure in which the heart is unable to pump enough blood to maintain the blood pressure and provide adequate nutrient flow to the internal organs.

We want to tell you more about broken heart syndrome, which is, unfortunately, a very, very real phenomenon—and illustrates vividly the tight link between a woman's emotional well-being and her heart health.

Scientists first became aware of this syndrome in the late 1990s. Heart specialists in Japan, then in Europe, and, ultimately, in the United States began to notice cases of women who had suffered an intense emotional stress (or sometimes a physical one) and appeared as though they were having a heart attack—but proved to have totally clean heart arteries.

These cases almost always were women rather than men. Usually, the affected women were post-menopausal. The emotional stress was always very severe—a breakup, an illness or the loss of a loved one, a devastating financial loss, diagnosis of a malignancy, or the like.

In such cases, a patient's EKG shows elevation of the ST segments, a surefire indication of a heart attack in evolution. The ST segments are a specific part of the tracing of an EKG of a single heartbeat and indicate active heart damage. The echocardiogram routinely reveals that the lowest half or two-thirds of the heart muscle has simply stopped pumping and is ballooning out instead of contracting with every heartbeat, as shown below.

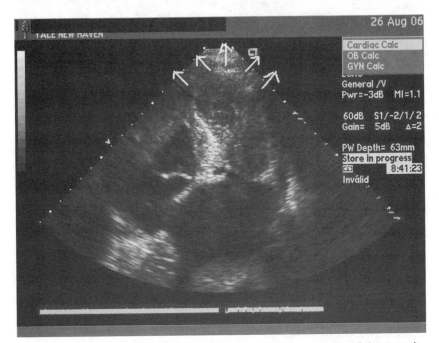

The echocardiogram in "broken heart" syndrome. Note the part of the pumping chamber of the heart (left ventricle) that "balloons" out instead of contracting. Arrows indicate direction of expansion of bulging rounded portion of left ventricle.

It is from that ballooning that the alternate name of the syndrome arises. In the United States, we call this the broken heart syndrome. In Japan, they call it "Tako-Tsubo" Syndrome. The word *Tako-Tsubo* refers to special, amphoralike clay pots that are used by fishermen to catch octopi.

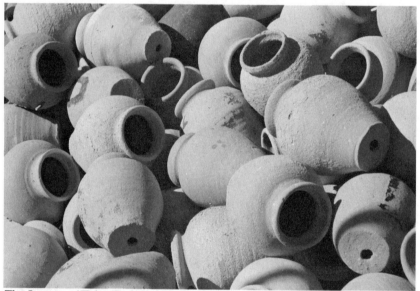

The Japanese "Tako-Tsubo" pots from which the "Broken Heart" syndrome gets its technical name. These pots trap the head of the octopus in the large, bulbous portion, so that the octopus cannot escape. The shape resembles the ballooning of the damaged part of the heart's pumping chamber in this syndrome. Photo courtesy of Stockxpert.com.

The pots are strung in line onto a rope extending from the boat to the bottom of the sea. The pots have a wide bottom and a narrow neck. The octopus squeezes his head into the pot, and is trapped, unable to extricate himself through the narrow neck. The rope is retrieved at the end of the day, the many amphoras laden with their valuable delicacies.

Although emotionally linked, the broken heart syndrome is absolutely, positively real. The EKG confirms a heart attack–type pattern. Blood tests show evidence of dead heart muscle cells. Images of the main pumping chamber of the heart display a large, nonfunctioning segment—like the wide bottom of the Tako-Tsubo pot. The patient develops heart failure (inadequate pumping strength of the heart). Powerful treatments are required—either drugs alone or a heart-assist device called a *balloon pump*.

Although broken heart syndrome patients are very sick—near death at times—complete recovery is the rule rather than the exception. (Maureen made a complete recovery and continues to be healthy to this day.)

To be frank, we do not have a clue as to how the emotional stress in broken heart syndrome leads to such severe, albeit transient, dysfunction of the heart. Scientists have postulated many potential links—via hormones, genetics, stress-related epinephrine release, even occult (undetected) or transient arterial blockage—but none has been conclusively shown to be the cause.

The simple fact is that the woman's heart is very complex, both physically and emotionally. Researchers still do not fully understand the links between the emotions and the physical manifestations in broken heart syndrome and in many other heart diseases, but there is much that we do know.

To convey the complexity of a woman's heart, as compared with a man's, is the prime reason why we have written this book for you.

This book will explore the many ways in which heart disease differs in women, with an eye toward helping you anticipate, recognize, and understand your heart better—so as to optimize your health and longevity.

# CHAPTER
# 1
# THE FEMALE HEART

## 1. NORMAL STRUCTURE AND FUNCTION

Your heart is a muscle, and a very special one at that. Just think about the simple fact that this muscle contracts every minute of every day for the entirety of your life. Can you imagine any other muscle in your body contracting continuously and without rest? Can you do pushups ad infinitum? How about situps? Not likely. Can you run continuously and indefinitely? Definitely not. Not even the world's best and most highly trained athletes can persuade any of their skeletal muscles (those that move the limbs) to work incessantly. Your heart muscle has unique innate cellular and metabolic traits that permit it to function continuously and without rest. No other muscle is tireless like your heart. (Your diaphragm is the only one that comes close, but the diaphragm is resting many of its fibers in rotation, except during peak exertion.)

For all this muscle activity, your heart needs blood flow and lots of it. A network of arteries on the surface of the heart—the coronary arteries—carries blood flow to the heart muscle itself. The oxygen and nutrients delivered to the heart muscle give your heart the energy to pump the blood within its chambers to the rest of the body. The word *coronary* refers to a corona, or crown. To early anatomists, the coronary artery network resembled a thin crown draped over the heart.

Figure 1.1 gives you an overview of the heart's anatomy.

**27**

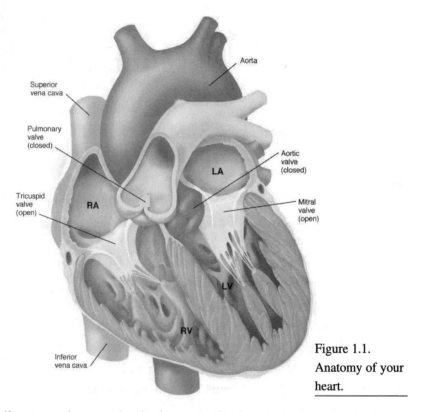

Figure 1.1.
Anatomy of your
heart.

Like any other mechanical pump, the heart needs valves to keep blood flowing forward. The pumping chambers of the heart need an inflow valve and an outflow valve. Without an inflow valve, blood already in the heart could leak backward, against the bloodstream. Without an outflow valve, blood already propelled forward would come right back to the heart. The proverbial Sisyphus of Greek mythology was cursed to push a heavy stone up a hill, only to start again when it rolled down. Without an outflow valve, the same would be true for your poor heart—there would be a heartful of blood pushed forward, only to have it come right back again, to be propelled once more.

The powerful pumping chamber of the heart is called the ventricle. The ventricle that pumps to your body is the *left* ventricle.

This blood goes to your head, your arms, your liver, your intestines, your legs, and virtually all organs of your body. The walls of the left ventricle are about one to two centimeters thick (about a half to one inch). This chamber pumps about five quarts of blood each and every minute. This requires an energy equivalent to about that used by an eighty-watt lightbulb. When an athlete is at peak exertion, his heart can pump ten or even twelve quarts of blood per minute.

You can follow the events of the cardiac cycle in figures 1.2a and 1.2b on page 30.

Leading into the left ventricle is the left atrium. The left atrium collects the blood coming back from the lungs and channels it into the powerful left ventricle. The left atrium, unlike the ventricle, is thin walled. It imparts only a small "boost" to the blood that it propels into the left ventricle. We liken the atrial chamber to the "turbocharger" of a high-performance car engine. It loads the main engine under pressure, thus improving its power output. The atrium boosts the output of your left ventricle by about one-fifth. The phase of the cardiac cycle during which the left ventricle is inactive, resting, and being loaded, is called diastole. It is the left ventricle that provides the powerful burst of squeezing action that propels the blood around the body. This phase of the cardiac cycle, when the left ventricle is contracting and ejecting blood, is called systole.

We have discussed only the left atrium and the left ventricle—the so-called left side of the heart. As you know, your heart also has a *right* side. The sole responsibility of the right side of the heart is to pump blood to the lungs. As you might imagine, this does not require as much power as is necessary on the left side of the body. Accordingly, the right ventricle is thin, about half a centimeter (or a quarter inch). It expends about twenty-watts of energy. The right ventricle has its own auxiliary atrium, called the right atrium, which boosts the blood entering the right ventricle. The right atrium

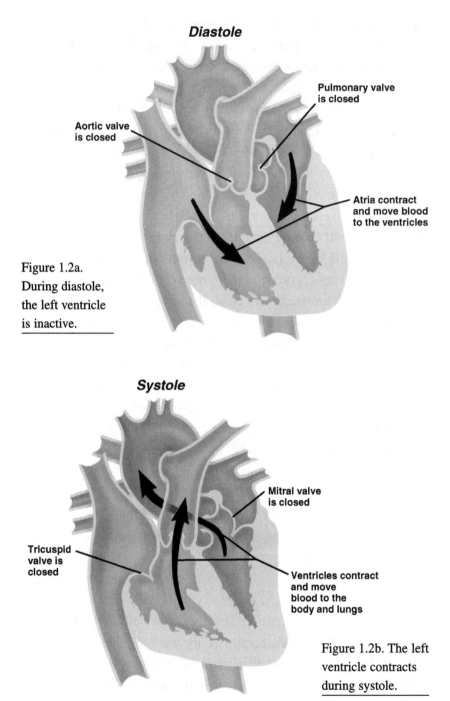

**Diastole**

Pulmonary valve
is closed

Aortic valve
is closed

Atria contract
and move blood
to the ventricles

Figure 1.2a.
During diastole,
the left ventricle
is inactive.

**Systole**

Mitral valve
is closed

Tricuspid
valve is
closed

Ventricles contract
and move
blood to the
body and lungs

Figure 1.2b. The left
ventricle contracts
during systole.

collects all the blood coming back from the body and channels it into the right ventricle, for delivery to the lungs.

So let's track a single drop of blood through your circulation. Let's pick it up on its way to a target organ, say, for example, your brain. (We could also pick any other organ or muscle in your body.) Under pressure from the heart, the drop of blood enters your brain and supplies the oxygen and nutrients to allow your brain to function—as in maintaining your consciousness and allowing you to read this book, for instance. After passing through your brain, the blood travels along the veins of your body back to the right atrium. The right atrium gives the drop of blood a little mechanical boost and channels it into the right ventricle. The right ventricle propels the droplet into your lungs, where it picks up oxygen from the air you breathe.

From your lungs, the drop of blood enters the left atrium, which gives it a boost into the left ventricle. The muscle-bound left ventricle—the main powerhouse of the heart—propels this drop of blood out again to your body, thus completing the never-ending circuit.

In general, patients with heart disease may experience some or all of the symptoms of the following types of heart problems: inadequate blood flow to the heart muscle (chest pain), congestive heart failure (shortness of breath), and arrhythmia, or altered rhythm, of the heart (severe lightheadedness or loss of consciousness). The most serious symptom of heart disease is cardiac arrest, which in earlier times was almost always lethal, and widespread access to defibrillators, but in this era of a highly educated public it is more often successfully treated.

## 2. ANATOMY AND PHYSIOLOGY OF A WOMAN— HOW THE FEMALE HEART DIFFERS

Your heart is smaller and lighter than a man's. A man's heart, on average, weight 177 grams (one third of a pound), while a woman's weighs only 118 grams (one quarter of a pound). Part of this difference is certainly because women are physically smaller than men. But the difference persists even if we take the body size into account. For example, if we calculate the mean weight of the heart for each sex and divide it by what we call the *body surface area* (a good index of body size), this should correct for any body-size differences. When we do this, we find that a man's heart weighs 92 grams for each square meter of body surface area and a woman's only 72. We can also compare the heart size with what we call *lean body mass*, or the amount of weight that would remain if all the fatty tissue disappeared. (This theoretical process would eliminate all the wonderful curves that make a woman a woman.) If this adjustment is approximated by special testing technologies, the woman's heart is just the same size as a man's, when compared with lean body mass.[1]

The smaller size of women's hearts makes us reluctant to use a female heart for transplantation in a male, whereas we are fine with placing a male heart into a female. (Still, one woman who received a male heart found herself suddenly drawn to beer and motorcycles; in fact, she wrote a book about her mental transformation. But such changes in personality have not been substantiated by any medical research. The larger and heavier male heart does not have any negative effects on women.)

Women have an advantage as they age, however. Their hearts do not lose muscle mass the way male hearts do. And as any cardiac surgeon knows, the female heart also has smaller coronary arteries which plays a role in the higher risk for women at the time of bypass or angioplasty (as discussed in the corresponding sections of this book). Bypassing these small arteries can pose a technical challenge.

## 3. CHANGES ASSOCIATED WITH PREGNANCY

Pregnancy most definitely has a major impact on the heart. The woman's circulatory system, by the end of pregnancy, is responsible for supplying blood and oxygen not only to a newly developing human being in her womb but also to the greater body mass of the woman herself. The amount of circulating blood nearly doubles by the end of pregnancy, doubling the heart's workload. The blood flow to the breasts increases, as does the blood flow to the uterus, from a trickle to more than a quart per minute. The blood flow to the skin increases by half, possibly as a means of dissipating heat. This strains a normal heart, let alone a diseased heart. If a woman has underlying heart disease, usually of the cardiac valves, the heart may be strained or fail during the course of pregnancy. The high blood pressure common in the last trimester of pregnancy puts an additional burden on the heart. The circulatory changes that accompany pregnancy are depicted in figure 1.3.

If you already know you have heart disease, you should have a consultation with a perinatologist as well as a cardiologist before getting pregnant. You will need to be followed closely by both physicians during pregnancy. Sometimes you do not know you have heart disease until the extra burden of pregnancy unmasks cardiac symptoms.

There are some heart diseases so serious that we advise you to avoid pregnancy if you suffer from them, such as cyanotic congenital heart disease, which refers to a congenital structural disease of the heart that renders your blood "blue" (that is, relatively devoid of oxygen). You should avoid or terminate a pregnancy if you have congestive heart failure (usually from a dilated heart) or if you suffer from pulmonary hypertension, which means "high pressure in the lungs."

Other, milder forms of heart disease mandate careful monitoring by a cardiologist during pregnancy but do not imply that pregnancy need be avoided or terminated—for example, a dilated heart with no accompanying symptoms or a narrowing of your aorta, called coarctation. You also need monitoring during pregnancy if you have had a valve replacement earlier in your life.

The testing of your heart is somewhat limited in preg-

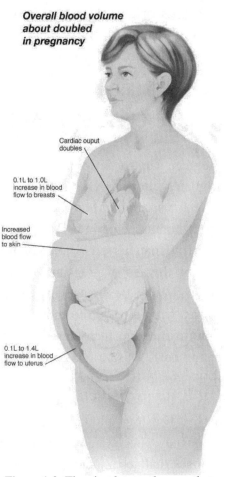

Figure 1.3. The circulatory changes that accompany pregnancy.

nancy because of the fetus. The fetus should never be exposed to the potential damaging influence of x-rays. Echocardiograms, however, are entirely safe. In fact, your baby likely has many echo exams through your abdominal wall even during the course of a normal pregnancy.

One very special and severe cardiac condition can occur during pregnancy—*aortic dissection* (see chapter 14). When this occurs related to pregnancy, it is called *peri-partum aortic dissection.*

Some patients with dilatation of the aorta may have an inherited condition characterized by a tall, thin body, which we call Marfan's syndrome. In women with an enlarged aorta, a tearing of the internal layers of the aorta can be brought on by the added circulatory burden of advanced pregnancy, by the high blood pressure of pregnancy, and especially by the dramatic straining and bearing down needed for childbirth. Most women affected by aortic dissection of pregnancy are made vulnerable by an underlying aortic enlargement or weakening. If you have a history of aneurysms or dissections in your family, please bring this to the attention of your obstetrician or perinatologist. Special precautions need to be taken. If your aorta is already dilated, we may recommend that you avoid or terminate pregnancy because the likelihood of aortic dissection may be too high. Fortunately, peri-partum aortic dissection is rare, but, when it does occur, it threatens both the mother and the baby.

If you are taking heart medications—such as antiarrhythmics, digoxin, diuretics, or blood pressure pills—these must be reviewed in detail with your doctor to determine if they are safe for the fetus.

The drug called Coumadin requires special attention.

## Can I Become Pregnant While Taking Coumadin?

Some young women do require an artificial heart valve and need to be treated with Coumadin. At times, these women have not completed their child-bearing years and want to become pregnant. This is somewhat difficult, but definitely possible.

First off, Coumadin itself is *not safe* for the baby and results in a high rate of miscarriage. Coumadin is what we call teratogenic, or damaging to the fetus—in fact, *highly so*. It is simply not appropriate to take Coumadin during your pregnancy, especially during the earlier phases.

So adjustments need to be made. Some women with an artificial heart valve can be carried through pregnancy without Coumadin, often with aspirin alone. More commonly, we substitute the drug heparin, which is not teratogenic, for Coumadin. Heparin and heparinlike drugs do not cross the placenta, so the fetus is not directly exposed to these drugs. The problem is that heparin cannot be taken orally—it is given by subcutaneous injection, just as insulin is injected by diabetics. This is not too onerous once you are used to it. An alternate form of heparin, known as Lovenox, can be given at more widely spaced intervals, so you should not need to give yourself a shot more than once, or at most twice, a day.

This whole process is safer if your artificial valve is in the aortic position, where it is relatively protected from clots. If your valve is in the mitral position, the risk of forming clots is higher. Still, with careful coordination between your obstetrician and your cardiologist, and a large measure of patience on your part, you can be carried through your pregnancy. The effort will all be worthwhile when your new baby is placed on your lap after delivery.

Because of these issues related to Coumadin, many young women opt for biological valves instead of mechanical valves (see chapter 11). Biological valves do not require blood thinners, and these Coumadin/pregnancy issues are thus obviated. However, the biological valve will wear out after about fifteen years, and another operation will be necessary.

# CHAPTER 2
# DISEASES OF THE HEART

**W**e've seen that your heart has blood vessels that give it nourishment. Inside your heart are intricate, delicate valves, which direct the flow through the various chambers of the heart. Your heart has an extraordinary electrical system that keeps its rhythm and rate regulated. And, of course, your heart is primarily a muscle, which gives *motive* force to the blood in your circulatory system.

We will now discuss what can go wrong with each of these major components—that is, how your heart can become diseased.

## 1. VESSELS—CORONARY ARTERY DISEASE

### Angina

The heart is a muscle. As such, it requires blood flow and oxygen delivery in order to function. In contrast to other muscles throughout the body, which function only episodically when needed, the heart pumps 24/7 throughout our lives. Even a period of seconds without heart function leads to unconsciousness and threat of organ damage. As noted earlier, the diaphragm, the large muscle of breathing that separates the chest from the abdomen, is the other muscle in the body that operates full-time, all the time. But unlike the heart, the diaphragm fires only a small fraction of its fibers with each contraction.

The heart's blood flow and oxygen requirements are huge. The coronary arteries, the small arteries that run on the surface of the heart, are about the size of the refill in your ballpoint pen (see figure 2.1). Their responsibility is to supply the nutrients the heart muscle needs. At rest, the heart requires about one cup of blood per minute to nourish itself. Under stress, it can utilize over one quart of blood per minute just to meets it own nutrient needs. This corresponds to about one-fifth of the total baseline flow of blood in the body.

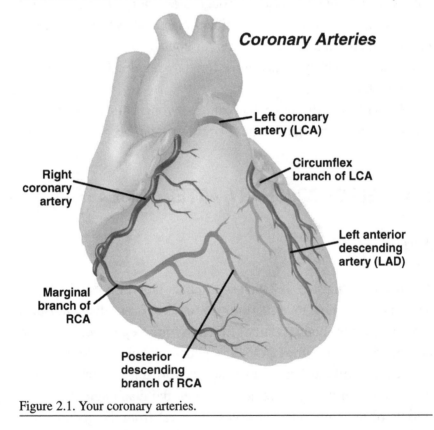

Figure 2.1. Your coronary arteries.

The coronary arteries originate directly above the aortic valve. There, two coronary arteries arise from the aorta and course over the heart like a crown, or corona, hence their name.

The left coronary artery bifurcates shortly after its beginning and becomes the left anterior descending and left circumflex coronary arteries. The former runs over the front surface of the heart, and the left circumflex coronary artery distributes itself over the lateral surface. The left anterior descending (or "LAD") coronary artery is by far the most important artery of the heart, by itself supplying over 40 percent of the total blood flow to the heart.

The other major coronary artery is the right coronary artery. In general, it supplies blood to the back surface of the heart.

Even a short interruption of blood flow to the heart muscle itself will lead to oxygen deprivation of the heart cells. This is felt as typical cardiac chest pain, or angina. The characteristics of this pain are that it is felt substernally, under the breastbone, and that it is perceived as a pressurelike pain. The classic scenario is that of a patient clutching her chest in severe discomfort (see figure 1 in the preface). The pain is often described in such terms as: "I feel like an elephant is sitting on my chest," or "I feel like I have a vise on my chest." The patient often uses a clenched fist over the chest to illustrate what she is feeling.

As we will see in chapter 5, a woman's symptoms often differ from those felt by a man. They may not be as typical and easily recognized as those we have just described.

Angina is actually the muscle burn that one can feel from any other muscle stressed to the point of exceeding its blood-flow capacity. For example, you can do situps to the point of exhaustion. The intense pain you will feel in your midsection is really "angina," so to speak, of your abdominal muscles.

We grade angina according to the level of exertion required to bring it on. This is called the Canadian Cardiovascular Society classification system. If the patient has no angina whatsoever, despite exertion, she is Class I. If angina comes on only with vigorous exertion (at the gym, for example), she is Class II. If the angina comes on with only mild exertion (as in walking on level ground), she is

Class III. If the angina comes on with no exertion, during the resting state, the angina is the highest category, or Class IV. Class IV patients may feel angina while resting, watching TV, reading, or even while sleeping.

Severe anginal attacks, especially those likely to eventuate in a heart attack, may be accompanied by profuse sweating. Friends or relatives may comment on an ashen color or an obvious appearance of physical distress.

Doctors used to think that all or most patients with inadequate blood flow to the heart would feel angina. We now know that many patients, perhaps up to 40 percent, do not. This may be dangerous for a number of reasons. First, these patients may escape diagnosis of their heart disease entirely. Second, even patients known to have heart disease may not be aware when they are exceeding their heart's capacity. After all, symptoms of disease, in general, reflect the body's intrinsic "early warning system." Patients who do not feel angina have a defective warning system.This is seen especially in diabetic patients (type 1 or type 2), in whom the sensory nerves are damaged by the excess ambient sugar levels in the body.

## The Role of Stress and Exertion

The root cause of angina arises from blockages in the coronary arteries, which supply oxygen-rich blood to the heart muscle itself. These blockages, as we shall see below, are caused by arteriosclerosis, or hardening, affecting the coronary arteries.

Classically, anginal pain comes on with exertion. The reason for this is that in the resting state, even with blockages in the arteries to the heart (see figure 2.2), the delivery of blood and oxygen is adequate to meet the heart's needs. As exertion proceeds, the heart needs more and more oxygen, and the blocked arteries cannot deliver. Patients often first notice heart pain, or angina, during bursts of severe exertion, such as running for a bus or hurrying between terminals at the airport.

Other states that can trigger angina, by increasing the heart's demand for oxygen above the available delivery, include stress and anxiety. For example, a patient may feel anginal discomfort during an intense marital dispute or during a stressful meeting at work.

Any activity that causes the heart to beat more rapidly or the blood pressure to rise may trigger angina. Oxygen demand may also exceed supply after a big meal, when blood and oxygen are diverted from the heart to the intestinal tract. An easy way to remember the major causes of angina is to think of the so-called three E's: exercise, emotion, and eating.

Characteristically, angina disappears when the exertion ends, as the demands for blood and oxygen come down to a level that can be met by the diseased arteries. Typically, angina goes away within a minute or two of sitting down and resting.

When pain comes on without any exertion or other provocation, we call that *angina at rest*. This is important because angina at rest may indicate that a heart attack is imminent. If you are getting chest pains when you are resting, seated comfortably, perhaps reading or watching TV, you have angina at rest. This is a potentially serious pattern, which you should call promptly to your doctor's attention.

## Coronary Artery Disease

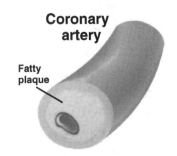

Coronary artery disease refers to the buildup of fatty deposits in the wall of one of the arteries that supply blood to the heart. This buildup narrows the central channel of

Figure 2.2. Buildup in the coronary artery.

the artery, decreasing the amount of blood and oxygen that can be carried to the heart muscle. Coronary artery plaques are composed of cholesterol fats, circulating cells from the bloodstream, and tissue cells reacting to the presence of all of these elements. The process of coronary arteriosclerosis takes decades to develop.

## Heart Attack

The process of arteriosclerosis occurs gradually, resulting in a pattern of regular angina. In some cases, a sudden adverse event sparks a heart attack. This plays out as follows.

If plaque ruptures into the central channel (or lumen) of a coronary artery, this material gets exposed to the bloodstream. The nature of this material causes clotting of blood that streams past it. As the blood clot (or thrombus) grows, it starts to block (or occlude) the coronary artery at the site of the plaque rupture. The expanding clot does not allow blood to flow by it, thereby depriving part of the heart muscle of blood and oxygen.

As this process extends into many minutes or hours, some of the heart muscle, deprived of oxygen, begins to die. Death of heart muscle is the definition of a heart attack. If blood flow is not promptly restored, the dead muscle is forever lost and forms a scar. We usually use the standard of four hours—if blood flow is not restored within this window of time, at least some of the affected muscle will die. This process is depicted in the figure 2.3.

The classical symptom of a heart attack is severe chest pain, which may be localized to the breastbone area or, in some patients, may radiate to the arms, shoulders, back, or jaw. Pain in the left arm is very common. Although the pain is often quite severe, there may be a number of variations. Pain may be intermittent or may be located in the upper abdomen. The pain may be rendered intermittent as the culprit clot may also undergo variable degrees of disso-

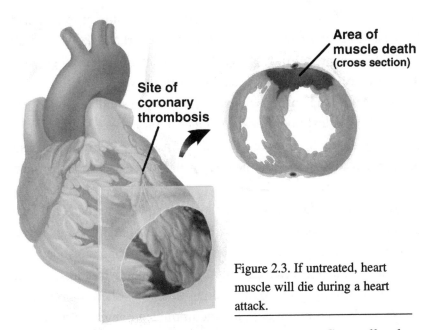

**Area of muscle death**
(cross section)

**Site of coronary thrombosis**

Figure 2.3. If untreated, heart muscle will die during a heart attack.

lution by the body's own reparative mechanisms. Generally, there is a feeling of significant weakness and a foreboding of doom. Sweating is common.

### Heart Attack or Angina Pain?

There are some distinguishing characteristics between an anginal episode and a heart attack. First and foremost is the duration. An anginal episode usually subsides within a few minutes. Beyond twenty minutes of pain is considered a heart attack in evolution—that is, the heart muscle cells have suffered from lack of oxygen long enough that at least some of them must be dying.

Another distinguishing characteristic is the relation to exertion. An anginal episode goes away when the exertion stops. Not so with a heart attack—the pain continues even after the exertion has stopped.

A third characteristic has to do with the response to a nitroglycerine tablet (TNG). An anginal episode will subside promptly with the first or second nitro tablet. Not so for a heart attack, whose pain continues despite nitroglycerine. The pain usually does not go away until you are given morphine in the hospital.

The pain of a heart attack usually comes on suddenly, reflecting the sudden occlusion (blockage) of a coronary artery. Anginal pain, on the other hand, is more gradual in onset, as exertion increases the oxygen demand of the heart muscle above what the coronary arteries can supply.

A patient having a heart attack may sense what we call "a feeling of impending doom," an intuitive sense that her life is in severe danger. This does not usually characterize an anginal episode.

A heart attack is often accompanied by other symptoms, such as nausea, vomiting, severe sweating, and an ashen complexion. These are less common with an uncomplicated anginal attack.

| *Some differences between an episode of angina and a heart attack.* | | |
|---|---|---|
| | **Angina** | **Heart attack** |
| Duration | 1 or 2 minutes | > 20 minutes |
| Relation to exertion | Subsides with cessation | Does not subside despite cessation |
| Response to TNG (nitroglycerine) | Responds well | Does not respond |
| Onset | Gradual | Sudden |
| Sense of doom | Not usually | Often |
| Associated symptoms and signs | Not usually | Nausea, vomiting, sweating, ashen color |

If in any doubt at all, you should dial 911 and be taken immediately to the hospital. The EKG will usually make it immediately clear whether you are experiencing a heart attack. (The EKG will also show whether you have suffered a prior major heart attack as well.)

A myriad other causes of chest pain are not due to a coronary artery problem. Gallbladder disease is a common alternative cause in women, as is hiatus hernia, where the upper portion of the stomach has situated itself above the diaphragm. Other causes of chest pain may be esophagitis, or esophageal spasm; a peptic ulcer; musculoskeletal pain or cervical spine disease; mitral valve prolapse; an inflammation of the lining surrounding the heart, or pericarditis; or states of anxiety. More serious causes of chest pain may include a blood clot to the lungs (a so-called pulmonary embolus), or a dissecting (splitting) aneurysm of the ascending aorta.

## Complications of a Heart Attack

| A Heart Attack Can Lead to a Variety of Complications ||
| --- | --- |
| COMPLICATION | COMMENTS |
| Ventricular tachycardia (regular but very rapid Ventricular fibrillation (chaotic, rapid rhythm) rhythm) | Very serious arrhythmias (usually cause cardiac arrest) |
| Heart block | Technical term for low heart rate |
| Heart failure | Decreased pumping strength due to muscle damage |
| Cardiogenic shock | Life-threatening decrease in pumping strength due to severe muscle damage |

| Mitral regurgitation | Leaking of the mitral valve (due to muscle damage near the mitral valve apparatus) |
| Embolization | Throwing off clots to other organs from the internal surface of the heart attack (brain is especially vulnerable) |
| Ventricular septal defect | Hole in the heart from internal "blow-out" between right and left ventricles |
| Cardiac rupture | "Blow-out" of the free wall of the heart |
| Pericarditis | Irritation of heart membranes by dead muscle |
| Death | May be the sequel to many of above complications |

A host of complications may ensue during the course of a heart attack and the early recovery. While this list is daunting, please keep in mind that the vast majority of heart-attack patients not only survive but also return to active lifestyles. The key is to get to the hospital early. Many complications can be prevented or lessened by immediate treatment. Even the most severe complications, like internal and external cardiac rupture, can be treated by surgery or other means.

Most patients who suffer a heart attack will go on to lead active, productive, and, in many cases, long lives. We are made with more heart muscle than we need. We can usually afford to lose a chunk or two without much discernible impact on lifestyle or capabilities or limitations. Yes, you will likely need to be on some medications or to have an angioplasty or even surgery. But unless your heart attack is extremely extensive, or you suffer multiple or repeated attacks, chances are that you will be able to carry on well with the activities of daily life.

## 2. VALVES—MITRAL VALVE DISEASE (INCLUDING MITRAL VALVE PROLAPSE), AORTIC VALVE DISEASE

As noted in chapter 1, the main pumping chamber of the heart—the left ventricle—has two main valves, an inflow valve called the mitral valve and an outflow valve called the aortic valve. Both are vital to the function of the heart, and both commonly become diseased in women.

Like valves in appliances or automobiles, the valves of your heart can be afflicted with one of two problems: narrowing (partial blockage), which is called stenosis, or leakage, which is called regurgitation or insufficiency.

Now, let's imagine the excess load that valve dysfunction would place on any pump. If the mitral valve is blocked, then blood cannot enter the left ventricle freely and easily. If the inflow valve is leaky, then blood will go *backward* through this valve when the heart contracts. You can easily picture that this cannot be good.

If the aortic valve is blocked, then blood cannot exit the heart freely and easily. It is almost as if your heart is being strangled. If the outflow valve is leaky, then blood propelled forward by cardiac contraction runs *backward* into the heart again. This also is very bad. Your poor heart is burdened like the mythologic character Sysiphus. As we mentioned in the introduction, this unfortunate character from Greek mythology was sentenced to roll a heavy rock up a large hill, only to have it roll back as soon as he reached the top. That is exactly the strain your heart suffers with a leaky valve; it has to pump the same blood over and over again out of your heart.

With these understandings, we have actually arrived at simple descriptions of the four conditions that can affect a woman's heart valves and potentially require surgery—aortic stenosis, mitral stenosis, aortic regurgitation, and mitral regurgitation. Let us now discuss each of these valve conditions, one by one.

## Mitral Stenosis

### Case Vignette: The Girl from Ipanema— Shock from a Tumor Blocking the Mitral Valve

Dr. Wackers, the distinguished and normally unflappable Dutch cardiologist, had grabbed Dr. Elefteriades by the lapel. The latter was about to leave town for a lecture trip. The morning's operation was complete and the patient safely ensconced in the ICU. Time was short to make the plane.

But Dr. Wackers would not take no for an answer. The patient was a twenty-three--year-old female from Brazil. She was living here with her husband, a graduate student in the business school. Sick for days, she had been shipped over to the univer-sity hospital from the infirmary. They thought she had mitral stenosis, narrowing of the mitral valve. So far, it sounded routine, hardly enough to cancel a major trip and justify the urgency of tone in the descriptions.

Then came more. The blood pressure was low, very low. Hmm, that wasn't right. The bicarbonate was five. Had Dr. Elefteriades heard right—five? No living patient could have a level so low, indicating extreme accumulation of acid in the body. The platelet count was 20, down from a normal 250. That could indicate only a premoribund condition.

Dr. Wackers took Dr. Elefteriades first to the echo lab. The minute the image came up on the screen, he knew his plans had to change. The tumor filled the left atrium, and each heartbeat blocked the mitral valve, virtually halting blood flow from the heart.

Orders were given to prepare the operating room, while the team hastened to the emergency room. From afar, Dr. Elefteriades saw a beautiful young woman, in full makeup and stylishly appointed. Only as the team got closer could he discern that she was barely breathing. No pulse was palpable anywhere, not in the arms, not in the neck, and not in the groin. Only with vigorous stimulation did Selma rouse to a momentary consciousness. The intern in the ER was dismayed that the doctor was not paying attention to the laundry list of laboratory parameters he was announcing—tests both completed and pending. Dr. Elefteriades had other plans. He grabbed the stretcher himself and started running for the elevator. The details of the labs did not really matter. The huge growth had to be removed. It was literally choking her heart to death.

Selma's tumor was removed successfully, and she recovered well. When last we heard from her, she and her husband were expecting their first child.

While Selma's case represents an extreme situation, it does illustrate how mitral stenosis can impair the heart's pumping function by blocking the mitral valve. Most cases of mitral stenosis, however, are caused not by a tumor but rather by rheumatic fever, a consequence of strep throat infection many years earlier. This, in turn, brings us to the next case vignette, concerning an old girlfriend of Dr. Elefteriades.

## Case Vignette: Rheumatic Fever: The Girlfriend

Dr. Elefteriades was just nineteen, a sophomore in college, when he met Angela. He was just getting to know her. They had had a great date, a fun ride back to her house in the convertible. Dr. Elefteriades was about to reach around her shoulder when he started to worry about that very "infectious" smile. Angela had told him she had suffered rheumatic fever when she was fourteen, losing two and a half months from school and gaining a heart murmur. She surely looked healthy now—very, very healthy, in fact. He was just about to kiss Angela, that all important first-kiss, when a little voice went off in his head. What is this rheumatic fever? Is it serious? Would it be done by now? Could it still linger? Was she in trouble? And, above all, was it contagious? In that era, kids didn't have AIDS to contend with, but mononucleosis was all the rage—the so-called kissing disease. Even then, young love had not been totally carefree. Angela leaned over, pursed her lips, and closed her eyes. Discretion was thrown to the wind. He decided to kiss first and ask questions later.

Little did Dr. Elefteriades know that years later, although rheumatic fever was definitely not contagious, its late ravages on the heart valves would form a substantial part of his cardiac surgical practice.

Mitral stenosis is the narrowing of the inflow valve of the left ventricle. It is almost always caused by rheumatic fever that occurred decades earlier. The rheumatic fever complicates occasional cases of strep throat. The strep throat goes away in a few days, but the effects of that original infection on the heart accumulate over years. The most common consequence is scarring of the tissue of the mitral valve leaflets, resulting in narrowing of the mitral valve, or mitral stenosis.

Mitral stenosis is largely a woman's disease, with a female preponderance of about three to one. Mitral stenosis puts a great strain on your lungs, as blood and pressure back up into the lungs because of the blockage in the mitral valve. You feel a lack of energy, as your heart is not able to pump enough blood due to the narrowing of the inflow valve to the left ventricle. Your left ventricle is protected and does not deteriorate over time, since it receives little load through the blocked mitral valve.

Figure 2.4 shows an example of mitral stenosis.

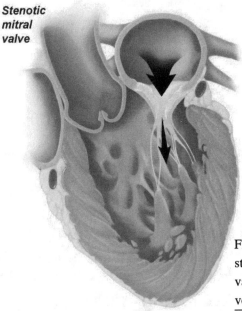

Stenotic
mitral
valve

Figure 2.4. In mitral stenosis, the mitral valve in the left ventricle narrows.

## Mitral Regurgitation

Mitral regurgitation is the leaking (backward) of the mitral valve. This is usually due to degeneration of the delicate structures that constitute your mitral valve and its supporting apparatus. The lungs become flooded by backward-leaking blood. The left ventricle is strained and often damaged by having to pump an excess of blood because so much blood leaks backward.

Figure 2.5 shows an example of mitral regurgitation.

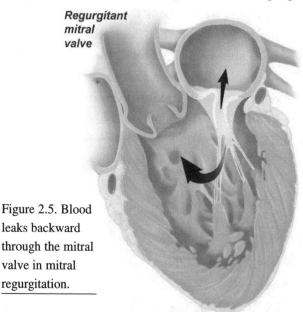

**Regurgitant mitral valve**

Figure 2.5. Blood leaks backward through the mitral valve in mitral regurgitation.

---

**Case Vignette: Recurrent "Anxiety Attacks" in a Young Woman**

Erica was a thin thirty-two year-old woman who was referred to me for evaluation by her primary care physician. The referring doctor was frustrated because the woman repeatedly presented to either his office or the emergency room with complaints of shortness of breath, irregular heartbeats, vague chest pain, and easy fatiga- bility. The primary care doctor and doctors in the ER were sure she was just having anxiety attacks and tried to reassure the patient, but she continued to present with the same symptoms. When I met Erica, she was exasperated and annoyed: "I am sure you will tell me the same thing as the rest of the doctors—I am just having anxiety attacks!" I told Erica I could understand why she felt that way. However, I wanted her to start from the beginning and describe all her symptoms—for how long, when they were more likely to occur, if there was any family history of heart problems, and her own use of medications, herbal products, and over-the-counter substances. Listening to the patient was very important and helped me determine the diagnosis. Erica's mother and an aunt had had "valve problems," and her aunt had required surgery to repair one of them. I proceeded with the physical exam and noted on her cardiac exam that Erica had a sound called a "click," as well as a soft murmur. I suspected Erica had mitral valve prolapse and ordered a test called an echocardiogram, which allows the heart muscle and valves to be viewed. Mitral valve prolapse was immediately confirmed and, in turn, explained all of Erica's symptoms.

Mitral valve prolapse (MVP) refers to a specific abnormality of the mitral valve leaflets that is particularly common in women. This condition involves a "floppiness" of the mitral valve so that one or both leaflets move excessively under pressure from the blood in the left ventricle during systole, or the active muscle contraction phase. Your doctor may hear a mild, short murmur or even a clicking sound through the stethoscope. In most cases, MVP occurs without any other heart disease, on its own, without any specific cause. There does appear to be a genetic component to this disease, and, if you have MVP, there is an increased likelihood that your siblings and children will also be affected. More than two-thirds of individuals with MVP are women.

Mitral valve prolapse can be asymptomatic, meaning that it produces no symptoms—in which case it is picked up during an

echocardiogram in an otherwise healthy woman. Mitral valve prolapse can also cause a variety of symptoms, including chest pain,
shortness of breath, palpitations, passing-out spells, and anxiety and
panic attacks. These symptoms are controversial, however, since
some individuals with anxiety and with or without MVP experience
the same symptoms.

MVP is quite common, seen in about 3 percent of human
beings. In most women with MVP, their outlook is fine—they will
feel well and live long. A small minority of MVP patients may be
prone to leakiness of the mitral valve and require mitral valve surgery on that basis. A few patients may be prone to sudden death, for
reasons that are not entirely clear. MVP tends to be more "benign,"
that is, milder, in women than in men. Unless you have a lot of
leakage of your MVP valve, it is likely that it will remain a
curiosity rather than a significant health issue for you. The leakage
usually does not progress markedly, and surgery is not frequently
necessary.

## Aortic Stenosis

Aortic stenosis is the narrowing of the aortic valve, the main outflow valve of your heart, causing a damaging lesion. This narrowing places a great strain on your heart, effectively choking it.
This usually occurs from "wear and tear" over seventy to eighty
years of life. When it happens in your forties, fifties, or sixties, it is
usually due to a congenital abnormality of the aortic valve, which
is called bicuspid aortic valve. Valves in such individuals have only
two leaflets instead of the normal three, and these valves wear out
easily and early (by middle age). Bicuspid aortic valve is very
common, affecting about 2 percent of the population.

Figure 2.6 shows an example of aortic stenosis. The buildup of
calcium is very common, exemplifying the "mechanical" nature of

valve disease. No medication in the world can remove the bonylike calcium deposits that have developed on this valve.

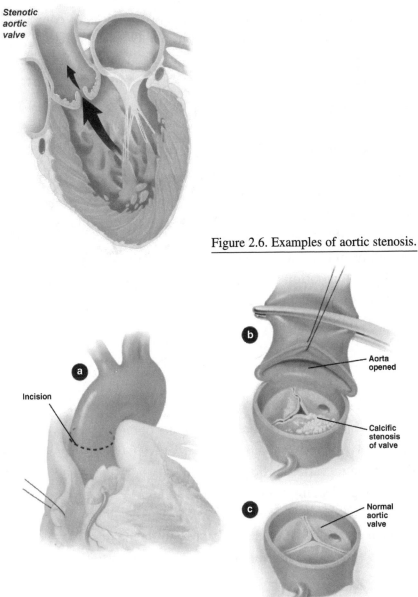

Figure 2.6. Examples of aortic stenosis.

Severe aortic stenosis can limit the amount of blood flow that the heart can pump. If you suddenly change position or abruptly exert yourself, the instantaneous demand for blood flow may exceed what the heart can actually deliver through your narrowed aortic valve. The net result is dizziness or even loss of consciousness because blood flow to the brain is inadequate. This is a very serious symptom of aortic stenosis.

## Aortic Regurgitation

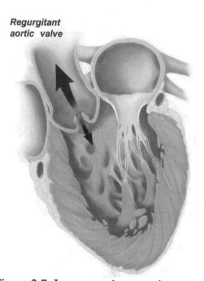

*Regurgitant aortic valve*

Aortic regurgitation is leaking of the aortic valve, forcing your heart to pump large volumes because so much blood leaks back into the heart after being ejected from the heart chambers.

The illustration shows an example of blood flowing backward through a leaky aortic valve.

Figure 2.7. In a regurgitant aortic valve, blood leaks backward.

♥ ♥ ♥

Valvular heart disease is one of the most common causes of heart failure. By the mechanisms indicated above (stenosis or regurgitation of the mitral or aortic valves), blood under pressure builds up in the lungs, leading to difficulty breathing. The heart enlarges, getting progressively weaker and weaker. This leads to fluid buildup throughout the body, most easily seen in the ankles. These constitute the explicit manifestations of congestive heart failure.

# 3. RHYTHM—IRREGULAR HEART RHYTHMS FREQUENTLY SEEN IN WOMEN

An arrhythmia is any abnormality of the basic heartbeat. The abnormality can involve the rate of the heart or the rhythm of the heartbeat. In arrhythmia, it is as if the tempo or syncopation of your heart's normal symphony has been disturbed.

Normally, the heart beats between sixty and a hundred times per minute. A heart rate less than sixty is called a sinus bradycardia (brady means "slow" in Greek), and a heart rate greater than a hundred is called a sinus tachycardia (tachy means "fast" in Greek). The term sinus is good. The sinus is the normal spot in the upper chamber of your heart where the heartbeat should originate. If the rhythm is initiated at a different site, the term sinus can no longer be applied, signifying a deviation from the norm.

A tachycardia that arises in the upper chamber, the atrium, is called an atrial tachycardia or atrial flutter. If the atrium is disorganized and does not initiate a regular rhythm, then the arrhythmia is likely atrial fibrillation. These rhythm disturbances arising from the upper chamber are generally not life threatening.

If the tachycardia is initiated in the lower chamber, the ventricle, then the rhythm is dangerous. Ventricular tachycardia, a life-threatening rhythm disturbance, often is a sign of severe underlying structural disease. The lower chambers have developed a rapid rate of their own, essentially like a runaway train. Ventricular fibrillation is the most dangerous rhythm disturbance and will lead to death if it persists for even a few minutes. In ventricular fibrillation, the heart muscle simply quivers, not even generating a single organized heartbeat.

You can get a sense of the aberrations and how they deleteriously transform a nice, normal sinus rhythm in the tracings presented in figure 2.8.

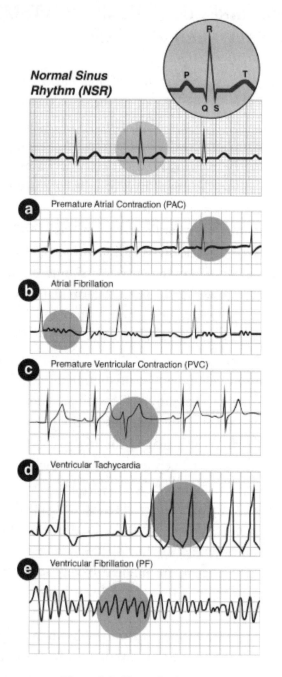

Figure 2.8. Heart rhythm tracings.

Very slow heart rates that do not arise in the sinus node are generally due to a condition termed heart block. In this condition, the atrium and ventricles lose their electrical connection and beat separately and independently. The intrinsic beat of the ventricle is usually slower than normal; hence, the heart rate is most often less than sixty beats per minute.

Ordinarily, people are unaware of their heartbeat. This is fortunate as the heart of an average person beats a half million times per week. Women who do feel an irregularity may describe their sensation in a variety of ways, such as a skip or a fluttering—like a bird beating its wings in the chest—or as a thumping, flip-flopping, or pounding in the chest or neck, or even as a tickle in the throat region. The most common form of palpitation is not due to heart disease but may simply be a heightened awareness of the heartbeat because of anxiety or tension.

Palpitations are most often due to a premature atrial or ventricular beat. The heart normally beats quite regularly, with each beat occurring at the same interval as the previous one. On occasion, even in a normal heart, an extra beat will occur prematurely, and the regularity of the rhythm will be disturbed. This premature beat will be followed by a heavy beat, as if the heart is trying to get caught up. This will be felt as an extra beat. Occasional extra heartbeats are entirely benign and very widespread among the population and different age groups.

Even in the absence of any heart disease, palpitations may be brought on by caffeine-containing beverages (coffee, tea, sodas), smoking, alcohol, emotions, or some prescription drugs used to treat asthma or other lung disorders.

Although most cardiac skips or arrhythmias are not serious, they should be brought to the attention of your physician.

Let's review how your physician may go about assessing your sense of irregular heartbeat. The history is sometimes a clue to the nature of an abnormal heart rhythm. Sudden onset or sudden cessation, regularity or irregularity, rapid or slow beat—these are helpful clues. At times, a simple test called an electrocardiogram will tell the story. But the electrocardiogram records less than one minute of the heart's action, and there are 1,440 minutes in a day. If the arrhythmia is present while the electrocardiogram is being taken, often no other investigation is necessary. The next step in unraveling the symptom is a test with a device called a Holter monitor, which records all the heartbeats over a twenty-four-hour period. Three or four small EKG pads are placed over the chest, and the data are sent to a tape recorder worn by the patient. The patient often also keeps a record of the times when any symptoms occur, which can then be correlated with what was happening with the heart's rhythm. The recording of these many, many heartbeats is interpreted by a specialist, with the aid of computerized analysis. This may pinpoint the abnormality, but often the patient may feel there is a symptom even though the electrocardiographic tape is perfectly normal.

If the EKG and Holter monitor are not helpful in pinpointing the problem, then the patient may be given an event recorder, which the patient usually keeps for a month. There is a continuous tape loop that erases itself after a built-in delay. If the patient senses a symptom, the electrocardiogram at that time can be transmitted telephonically and recorded at the monitoring center. Since arrhythmias are often random, intermittent, and infrequent, the event recorder can be helpful in identifying the underlying abnormal heart rhythm that is causing symptoms.

Lastly, the most sophisticated technique available for identifying an arrhythmia is called an EP test, or electrophysiologic testing. This is a technique in which a catheter is placed in the atrium or ventricle and electrical stimulation is given to the heart. The goal is to identify the type of arrhythmia that is causing the trouble—by provoking the abnormal rhythm electrically. The EP test is highly effective in predicting your susceptibility to future serious arrhythmic events. If the test is negative—your heart cannot be tickled electrically into a serious arrhythmia—the outlook for your arrhythmia is very good. If, on the other hand, your arrhythmia is easily induced during the EP test, chances are very high that you will have a serious arrhythmia during your normal daily activities. In such a case, some treatment may be recommended, with drugs, by catheter, or even by surgery.

The description of the EP test probably sounds troublesome to you. But, believe it or not, this type of test is very safe. Patients almost always survive the procedure itself free of major adverse consequences during or after such testing. Yes, you may—and probably will—need to be defibrillated during the course of this test, but, in this setting, that is routine. The doctors are specially trained and skilled at recognition and management of these serious rhythm abnormalities. The information will be of great importance for your future safety. In addition, you will be sedated appropriately, and chances are you will have no discomfort or recollection.

For some women, a *slow* rather than a *fast* heart rate might be the problem. In many cases, the slow heart rate is caused by the wear and tear of aging. The spot of tissue in the right atrium that normally initiates the heartbeat—called the sinus node—may become "tired" with age and fail in its function. Or the "wires" that normally transmit the electrical impulse throughout your heart muscle may become dysfunctional with age. In fact, these "wires" are actually made of nerve cells, which degenerate with aging.

In other cases, a heart attack may kill important nerve cells, just like it affects the heart muscle itself. In such a case, a slow heart rate results. This will give you a very slow pulse, which you can feel at your wrist or in your neck. This is different from the normally slow pulse that healthy athletes often have, reflecting their high state of conditioning.

Rarely, heart block may be caused by an internal infection within the heart. Lyme disease rampant in the Northeast, is one potential such cause of heart block, even (and especially) among young individuals.

The conduction system of the heart, its "electrical wiring," so to speak, is truly remarkable. The sinus node initiates the signal that triggers a heartbeat. The electrical wave spreads over the atria to a second specialized tissue called the atrio-ventricular node. From there the conduction wave enters the ventricles through channels called the left and right bundle branches. As the electrical wave activates the ventricular muscle, the ventricles contract, ejecting blood respectively into the lungs from the right ventricle and into the aorta from the left ventricle. Over the course of a lifetime, the electrical system activates the heart over two billion times. It is a remarkable system in that even a four- or five-second failure would lead to a state where unconsciousness, and even death, might occur.

It is when the conduction system starts to falter, usually after many decades of continuous activity, that a cardiac pacemaker may be required.

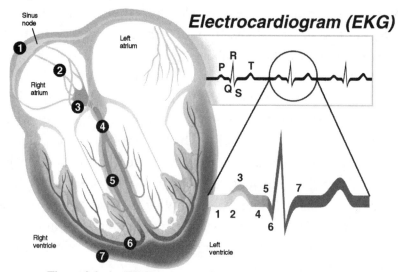

Figure 2.9. An EKG measures the heart's electrical activity.

Some women, especially those with disease of the sinus node or the remainder of the conducting system, may actually faint because of the electrical problem with the heart. The medical word for fainting is syncope. Fainting usually results after the brain has been deprived of oxygen and blood for about ten seconds. Fainting is often caused by electrical problems like those we are discussing in this chapter; however, other noncardiac causes exist as well, including diseases of the brain and a variety of abnormalities of the arteries and veins that secondarily cause inadequate blood flow to the brain.

Fainting that occurs during exercise or directly thereafter is often cardiac in origin. It may be due to a ventricular arrhythmia precipitated by inadequate coronary blood flow during exercise. It may also reflect one of two conditions representing obstruction to the flow of blood as it leaves the heart: valvular narrowing, called aortic valve stenosis, or a muscular narrowing, called hypertrophic cardiomyopathy with obstruction.

Fainting may also occur due to complete heart block, where the rate of the heart cannot increase enough to keep the brain oxygenated. At times very rapid heart rates may lead to syncope, as the heart does not have sufficient time between beats to fill in preparation for the next ejection.

Syncope can be due to an obstruction in the blood vessels in the neck that carry blood and oxygen to the brain, the carotid arteries. See figure 2.10. Severe narrowing may limit blood flow through them to the brain. This can be treated by a surgical procedure that removes the offending deposits and restores unimpeded blood flow.

Sometimes fainting may be mediated through the nervous system. The vagus nerve, when stimulated, slows the heart rate. In certain individuals, severe emotion may activate the vagus, leading to profound slowing of the heart rate and fainting. The classical Victorian faint is of such variety. Fainting at the sight of blood is probably another example. These types of faint are usually not terribly serious.

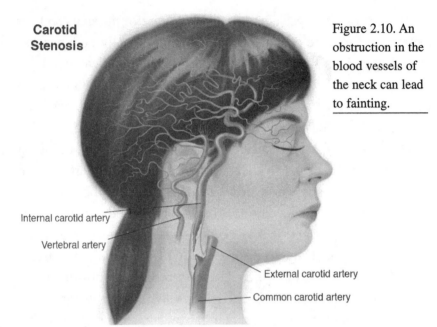

**Carotid Stenosis**

Figure 2.10. An obstruction in the blood vessels of the neck can lead to fainting.

Internal carotid artery

Vertebral artery

External carotid artery

Common carotid artery

Lastly, there exists a collection of nerves within the neck called the carotid sinus. In the presence of an overactive carotid sinus, the vagus nerve can be activated excessively, leading to a drop in heart rate. Turning the head in one direction or another or bending the neck may activate the carotid sinus and lead to fainting from too slow a pulse. This syndrome can be mild or serious, depending on severity and frequency of fainting.

## Causes of fainting

Slow heart rate
Carotid artery narrowing
Cardiac arrhythmias
Aortic valve stenosis
During urination
    (micturition syncope)
Hypertrophic obstructive
    cardiomyopathy

After cough (cough syncope)
Low blood pressure
Epilepsy
Vasovagal syncope (Victorian
    swoon) (anxiety, fright)
Allergic reaction
    (bee sting, or other)
Dehydration

## Atrial fibrillation

Atrial fibrillation is so common in women that we should discuss this in some detail. In certain cases, we can identify specific causes of atrial fibrillation. For example, the strain of a blocked mitral valve, called mitral stenosis, can cause the left atrium to struggle, enlarge, and lapse into atrial fibrillation. In most cases, however, atrial fibrillation is just due to aging and wear and tear on the heart. In fact, up to 15 percent of patients over eighty have had atrial fibrillation at some point.

### Case Vignette: The Doctor's Mom and Her Fluttering Heart

The atrial fibrillation was driving her mother crazy, Dr. Martha Matthews was telling one of the authors on the phone. Martha was a doctor, an ophthalmologist, but she admitted to knowing almost nothing about the heart. "That's about as much as I know about the eye," the author thought.

Mom was seventy-eight. She had been in very good health. Two months before, she had developed atrial fibrillation, an "arrhythmia," or abnormal heart rhythm, to which the elderly are especially prone. In this arrhythmia, the upper chambers of the heart contract at a very rapid rate (often up to 180 beats per minute or more) and in a very irregular pattern. That was exactly why Mrs. Matthews felt the rapid fluttering, or palpitations, in her chest. She didn't like it one bit. It just didn't feel right. It felt dangerous. She wanted to do something—move, cough, drink some water—but nothing made it feel better.

Dr. Matthews explained that her mother's energy was down dramatically since the atrial fibrillation had come on. That was not surprising, as the loss of slow, regular contraction of the upper chambers robbed the heart of 15 to 20 percent of its output.

And the medications, what a burden they were to Mrs. Matthews, her daughter explained. There were the antiarrhythmics, aimed at restoring a normal pattern of heartbeat. Then, there were the blocking drugs, the ones meant to bring the heart rate down from the stratosphere. And, above all, those blood thinners were troublesome. The family doctor had explained that, with the atrial fibrillation, Mrs. Matthews was at risk for developing clots in the heart—clots that could travel to the brain and cause a stroke. Stroke was a word Mrs. Matthews had not wanted to hear. She had seen too many of her elderly friends go down that path.

So, Dr. Matthews explained, Mom liked nothing about this new atrial fibrillation. Wasn't there something we could do about it? Couldn't we set it right again—with meds or electrical paddles or something?

A visit was scheduled, and we looked forward to meeting Mrs. Matthews and fine-tuning her cardiac care.

Sometimes, drugs or electrical conversion may restore a sustained normal rhythm. Unfortunately, the atrial fibrillation often will be permanent. In such a case, controlling the overall heart rate with drugs diminishes the subjective sensations felt by the patient. The rhythm is still technically atrial fibrillation, but with the racing heart rate now controlled, the patient is not as cognizant of the aberration. Many elderly patients cease to be aware of the arrhythmia entirely, essentially becoming used to it.

Currently, there is great deal of enthusiasm for trying to eliminate atrial fibrillation with a catheter-based procedure (called an ablation) or a minimally invasive operation (sometimes called a mini-Maze). These procedures can be very effective in certain patients, eliminating the atrial fibrillation completely and permanently. Since the patients likely to have a good response cannot readily be identified, you should be aware that the overall effectiveness of these procedures is as yet unclear. Many patients continue to have atrial fibrillation, still need drugs, and still need to undergo periodic electrical cardioversions. If you are interested, you should discuss this procedure fully with your cardiologist and your cardiothoracic surgeon.

## 4. MUSCLE—CAUSES FOR HEART MUSCLE FAILURE

The muscle of your heart is the actual motivator for the propulsion of blood. The arteries, valves, and conducting system of your heart that we have just discussed are useless without the actual muscle of the heart. Fortunately, the heart muscle is robust and usually works for a lifetime without deterioration. However, it is susceptible to damage from various causes, potentially leading to heart failure or insufficient ability of the heart to circulate your blood. These causes include:

1. *Heart attack.* The heart muscle can be damaged by a heart attack. The meaning of heart attack, technically called myocardial infarction, is death of a part of the heart muscle. This is far and away the leading cause of heart muscle damage.
2. *Valve disease.* The valvular lesions we discussed above can put a strain on the heart muscle, by way of pressure (aortic stenosis) or volume overload (aortic or mitral regurgitation). Over months to years, this strain can lead to actual weakening of the heart muscle. This may be partially, but not fully, reversible by corrective valve surgery.

## Case Vignette: The Lovely Lady with the Failing Heart

A sweet, previously healthy mother of four with a loving husband was admitted urgently in transfer from another hospital in what is called "cardiogenic shock." Cardiogenic shock represents the most severe, advanced state of inadequate pumping by the heart. The heart contractions are so weak that there is not enough blood flow to keep the body's organs functioning. The blood pressure falls very low; the kidneys stop making urine; and the patient usually succumbs in short order if drastic measures are not taken.

We took Angie directly to the operating room. We put in one type of artificial heart to replace the function of the left side of her heart and another to replace the function of the right side. She remained very sick for days but eventually started making steady progress. When she resumed consciousness and was weaned from the breathing machine, her first comment had to do with what a "racket" the noisy mechanical heart devices made inside her body.

One never knows, but some such cases of heart failure are caused by viruses that eventually clear from the body (see below). This seemed to be the case with Angie. Not only did she improve with the artificial hearts pumping loads of blood to her organs, but her own heart started to make blips in her blood pressure tracings—it was coming to life again. In several weeks, we removed the right-sided artificial heart. With continued improvement of Angie's own heart, a week later, we removed the left-sided artificial heart. She was now on her own! Her so-called viral cardiomyopathy (weakness of the heart muscle due to viral infection) had cleared. She was discharged to her family in good condition. She just sent a picture of a very healthy young woman running around the yard with children and husband—herself, looking like she had never been sick.

3. *Viral infection.* Most of us suffer from a cold, a virus, or the flu once or more per year. For most of us, these viral infections come and go, with some transient symptoms, but no permanent sequeallae (the medical term for "consequences"). For a very small, unfortunate minority, the virus can take hold of the heart muscle, surreptitiously damaging its cells. Heart failure can eventuate, often not until months or years have passed in the unsuspecting affected individual. Fortunately, only a very, very minute fraction of viral illnesses result in any heart damage.

4. *Infiltrative diseases.* Systemic diseases (that is, those that affect the whole body) can also affect the heart muscle. This is the case with amyloid, sarcoid, and a number of other chronic diseases that infiltrate multiple body organs.

5. *Hypertrophy.* Muscle hypertrophy is a Greek word for "muscle bound." Now, a muscle-bound state may be good for your biceps or your quadriceps—so-called skeletal muscles because they are responsible for moving your skeleton and the body it supports—but it is not good at all for your heart. A hypertrophied heart is stiff and unsuitable for its pumping function. The heart can become hypertrophied from an inherited disorder or from chronic hypertension. The strain of pumping against a high pressure in the arteries leads the muscle to thicken and stiffen, in the way that your biceps will thicken and stiffen if you do weight curls every day.

6. *Toxicity.* Certain exogenous substances and drugs can actually damage the heart muscle cells and lead to inadequate pumping strength of the heart. This is the case with alcohol consumed in large quantities over a sustained period of time. Alcohol-induced heart muscle weakness is quite common. This can revert, at least partially, after a period of abstinence.

(A small daily intake of alcohol, especially red wine, can actually be good for the heart. It takes more severe and sustained drinking to cause the heart damage referred to in this section.) Certain chemotherapeutic agents, used for the treatment of Hodgkin's disease or other malignant conditions, can lead to heart muscle weakness; this is especially true for the drug Adriamycin.

7. *Idiopathic*. *Idiopathic* is another Greek word incorporated into medical parlance, which means "coming of its own accord." This describes a medical condition for which medical science simply does not know a cause. Many cases of heart failure are idiopathic—more often than you would expect.

When the heart muscle is weakened by any of the above processes, the forward flow of blood is impaired, leading to light-headedness and weakness. Blood backs up in the lungs because it is not adequately propelled forward, resulting in a feeling of congestion and shortness of breath.

Medications or surgery can be used to correct heart failure. Ultimately, if necessary, you may need to have a mechanical heart or a heart transplant.

# CHAPTER
# 3
# PHASES OF A WOMAN'S LIFE: WHAT ARE THE HEART RISKS?

## 1. YOUNGER THAN FORTY-FIVE: THE "HONEYMOON" PERIOD

Heart disease most commonly occurs in both men and women over the age of forty-five. However, younger men and women can develop heart disease and have heart attacks. Women who have heart attacks at a young age usually have several risk factors for heart disease.

*Tobacco.* Studies have shown 65 to 92 percent of patients who have heart attacks under the age of forty smoke cigarettes. The risk of having a heart attack is increased sixfold in women who smoke twenty cigarettes per day, compared with women who do not smoke.[1] If there is only one thing a woman can do for her health, it is to stop smoking!

*Family history.* Younger women with heart disease more often have a family history of premature heart disease. The largest study examining this link found that 64 percent of young patients with heart disease had a family history of it.[2] It is important to discuss your family history with your doctor. If you go to the emergency room with possible symptoms of a heart attack, make sure you tell the doctor who's evaluating you if your parents or siblings have heart disease.

*Cholesterol.* Abnormalities in the cholesterol levels are very common in young women with heart disease. The most frequent are high triglyceride (one type of bad cholesterol) and low HDL (good cholesterol) levels.[3] All women should have their cholesterols checked by the age of twenty; if the cholesterol levels are normal, the tests should be repeated every five years. If you have a very strong family history of heart disease (parents with heart disease at a young age, a brother or sister with heart disease), or a known family history of cholesterol problems, cholesterol levels should be evaluated at a younger age.

*Obesity.* Obesity is recognized by the American Heart Association as an independent risk factor for heart disease.[4] In the United States, 23.3 percent of women between the ages of twenty to twenty-nine are obese, and 32.5 percent of women between the ages of thirty to thirty-nine are obese.[5] Obesity is also associated with the development of traditional risk factors such as high blood pressure, diabetes, and abnormal cholesterol levels. Regular daily exercise and proper nutrition should start in childhood because if you are overweight or obese as a child, you are more likely to struggle with obesity as an adult. Unfortunately, very few of us exercise three or more times per week as is recommended by the American Heart Association as is shown in figure 3.1.

**Figure 3.1. Percentages of Americans with Various Exercising Habits**

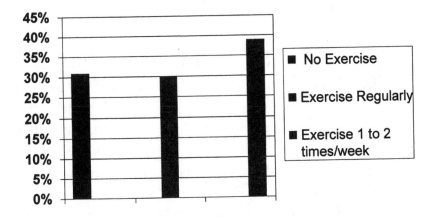

*Drugs*. Cocaine has been associated with 25 percent of heart attacks in patients between eighteen and forty-five.[6] Cocaine constricts the arteries that provide nutrient blood flow to your heart muscle. It may seem harmless to try drugs when you are young, but there are serious risks to your heart. Severe damage to the heart muscle as a result of a heart attack can happen with the use of cocaine. Is it worth risking your life and the ability to run and play with your children in the future?

*Pregnancy*. Heart attacks are rare in young women, although the risk is increased during pregnancy, usually during the last trimester and in the early postpartum period. In a recent report of pregnancies between 2000 and 2002 in hospitals in the United States, 859 discharges from the hospital included a diagnosis of heart attack.[7] The three risk factors listed below have been shown to be associated with an increased risk of a heart attack with pregnancy:

- Age greater than thirty-five
- High blood pressure
- Diabetes

If you are a woman with one or more of these risk factors you should consult with a perinatologist (a doctor specializing in high-risk pregnancies) if you are considering getting pregnant.

## 2. AGES FORTY-FIVE TO SIXTY-FIVE: THE BEGINNING OF CHANGE AND MENOPAUSE

*Menopause.* Menopause is officially defined as the last menstrual flow. The perimenopause is the two years or so preceding this event. Menopause and perimenopause are correlated with decreased estrogen levels. Estrogen in premenopausal women keeps the HDL (good cholesterol) level high and relaxes the blood vessels. This beneficial effect is decreased after menopause. However, it is not menopause that puts a woman at significant risk for developing heart disease; it is the number and severity of untreated risk factors. As you approach menopause, be aware of your risk factors for heart disease and be proactive in discussions with your healthcare provider about treatment options to keep your heart healthy.

*Obesity.* Forty-one percent of women between fifty and fifty-nine years of age are obese.[8] In middle-aged and older women, obesity is associated with heart disease and the development of other risk factors for heart disease. Regular exercise and proper nutrition, with attention to portion size, will help control weight. It is very easy to gain two pounds a year as you age. That may not seem like much when you are twenty-eight years old, but if that continues for twenty years, you will find yourself a forty-eight-year-old trying to lose forty pounds. It can be hard to get started on an exercise program.

## RATE OF PERCEIVED EXERTION

During exercise, use the RPE (Rate of Perceived Exertion) Chart to monitor how you are feeling.

Try to achieve an RPE of 11 to 15 during exercise.

Do not exercise above an RPE of 15.

| RPE: Rate of Perceived Exertion | | |
|---|---|---|
| Rate how you feel overall during exercise. Take into consideration your muscles, breathing, and overall exertion. | | |
| 6<br>7<br>8<br>9<br>10 | Very, Very Light<br><br>Very Light | Warm-ups or Cool-downs |
| 11<br>12<br>13<br>14<br>15 | Fairly Light<br><br>Somewhat Hard<br><br>Hard | Just Right |
| 16<br>17<br>18<br>19<br>20 | Very Hard<br><br>Very, Very Hard | Slow Down!! |

## A Typical Aerobic Workout

| | Warm up | Aerobic | Cool down |
|---|---|---|---|
| Why? | Slow increases in HR and BP help to prevent injury | Experience main benefits of exercise | Slow decrease in HR and BP, reduces soreness |
| How? | Calisthenics, stretching, machines | Machines, aerobics, walking | Calisthenics, stretching, machines |
| How Long? | 5 to 10 Minutes | 20 to 60 minutes | 5 to 10 minutes |
| How Hard? | Light | Somewhat hard | Light |

*High blood pressure.* We generally consider pressure readings above 140/90 to represent hypertension (high blood pressure), often thought of as a condition that doesn't impact women. That is not true, especially once women reach menopause. After women lose the protection of estrogen at the time of menopause, the incidence of high blood pressure increases. As estrogen levels decline, arteries lose some of their ability to relax. At your annual physical exam, you should ask what your blood pressure is and how it compares with previous readings. High blood pressure places you at high risk for stroke, heart attack, and kidney failure. Healthy lifestyles such as regular exercise, weight management, and a low-salt diet all help decrease your risk of developing high blood pressure.

## 3. OLDER THAN SIXTY-FIVE: AGING AND THE FEMALE HEART

Your risk of developing heart disease increases significantly with age. The proportion of deaths due to heart disease in older women is 56 percent, while fewer than 20 percent of women's deaths in this age group are from cancer.[9]

*High blood pressure.* High blood pressure is one of the most common problems in older women and puts them at risk for heart disease as well as stroke. In fact, 70 to 80 percent of women over the age of seventy have high blood pressure.[10] High blood pressure should be treated with lifestyle modifications, including diet, exercise, and weight management as well as with medications. Just because you are an older woman does not mean you should not be treated for your hypertension, so as to decrease your risks for heart attack and stroke.

*Cholesterol.* The LDL (bad cholesterol) levels in women increase after menopause and are equal to those of their male peers between the ages of fifty-five to sixty. However in the older age groups, women's LDL cholesterol levels are even higher than those of men. Just as men get treated for cholesterol, so should women. It is important to know your cholesterol numbers and talk to your doctor about the recommended goals to decrease your risk of heart disease.

*Diabetes.* Rates for adult-onset diabetes increase as you age. The overall prevalence of diabetes is over 10 percent in people over the age of sixty-five. Heart disease is the leading cause of death in elderly patients with diabetes; risk-factor reduction is very important for all women who fall into this category.[11] This includes medications to control the glucose levels, treatment of high blood pressure and cholesterol, regular exercise, and taking an aspirin each day (if you're not allergic to it).

*Depression.* Depression is common in the elderly, especially those with diabetes, and can lead to the progression of heart disease. Women should feel comfortable talking about symptoms of depression with their doctors and getting appropriate treatment and support. Depression is in and of itself a very strong risk factor for heart disease and cardiac events.[12]

In summary, a great deal is known about heart disease at the different phases of your lifecycle. Many therapies and lifestyle modifications are available to decrease risk factors and should be a high priority for every woman:

- Stop smoking, particularly among young women.
- Moderate your use of alcohol: one drink per day.

- Maintain proper nutrition and weight management.
- Engage in regular physical activity at all ages.

# 4

# ARE YOU A WOMAN AT RISK FOR HEART DISEASE?

## 1. DOES AGE IMPACT YOUR RISK?

*Every woman needs to be evaluated for her risk of heart disease.*

Sara arrived at the emergency department complaining of chest pain radiating to her neck and back for over twelve hours. When the doctors evaluated her and told her and her family she had had a heart attack, they did not believe them. How could she have a heart attack when she was only forty-five years-old? Heart attacks, she thought, only happened to older people, right? Sara went for routine physical examinations each year, but her doctor never talked to her about heart disease.

Heart attack and stroke, as noted earlier, are the leading causes of death in women, responsible for more deaths each year than all other causes combined including breast cancer.[1] In fact, more women die from heart attacks each year, compared with men. The risk of a woman having a heart attack increases after menopause, due in part to increasing age but also to the presence of risk factors for heart disease (that we will review below). The older a woman gets, the more likely she is to get heart disease. Coronary heart disease is less common in premenopausal women, especially if there is no family history of heart disease and no other risk factors. A family tendency to heart disease is especially evidenced in a father affected before the age of fifty-five, a mother affected before the age of sixty-five, and coronary heart disease in a sibling. In general, younger women who have heart attacks have multiple cardiac risk factors, usually including smoking and often a family history of the disease. However, if you do have a positive family history, even strongly so, there is no need to despair. Many risk factors are related to lifestyle and can be modified, and drugs to control your risk factors can be highly effective. Women of all ages should be knowledgeable about heart disease and its risk factors and should take steps toward its prevention.

## 2. DO RACE AND ETHNICITY IMPACT YOUR RISK?

Linda is a postmenopausal sixty-five year-old grandmother of three and active in multiple community projects. She called her doctor today because she heard on the radio that being an African American woman puts her at greater risk for having a heart attack. Linda is overweight and has been told by parish nurses that her blood pressure is high, but she attributes this to being "nervous" when she gets her blood pressure taken.

Race is an important risk factor for developing heart disease, especially for African American and Hispanic women, who have a substantially greater risk of developing heart disease when compared with women of other races and ethnicities. One reason is the greater number of risk factors present in African American and Hispanic women, such as high blood pressure, lack of physical activity, obesity or overweight state, poor nutrition, and diabetes. Statistics from the Centers for Disease Control and Prevention on important risk factors in African American women are telling.[2] Over 46.6 percent of African American women have high blood pressure; over 51 percent are obese; 54 percent have high cholesterol levels; and almost twice as many have diabetes, compared with Caucasian women. The greater the number of risk factors, the greater the risk of heart attack and stroke in women of all races. According to the American Heart Association, 53.5 percent of African American women die from cardiovascular disease, compared with 35 percent of Caucasian women.

Unfortunately, many women of color are not appropriately informed and screened for risk factors. One of the most important ways to stop heart disease in women of all races is to improve education and awareness about the causes of heart disease and the actions both women and their doctors need to take. The following cases will illustrate the risk factors and the role each plays in increasing the likelihood of heart disease.

## 3. HOW DOES FAMILY HISTORY AFFECT YOUR RISK?

Kathy is a forty-year-old woman who has been in good health. However, she received a call from her brother's wife to say he had just been admitted to the hospital after having a heart attack. He was lucky. He'd arrived at the hospital within one hour of the onset of symptoms and had a stent placed in a vessel to his heart. Her brother is a forty-two-year-old non-smoker in good health who went to the doctor only every two to three years.

It is essential to know your family history and be sure to give this information to your healthcare provider. Several scientific studies have examined the role of family history and its impact on the risk of developing coronary heart disease. Younger patients with heart disease often have a family history of premature heart disease, such as a father younger than fifty-five or a mother younger than sixty-five having been diagnosed with heart disease. Family history is a strong predictor of developing heart disease even more commonly in women than in men. In addition to showing a link to parents with heart disease, the Framingham Offspring Study demonstrated the important finding that heart disease in a sibling was also associated with a significant increase in risk for the development of heart disease.[3]

The American Cancer Society has done a great job in educating women on their risk of breast cancer and the importance of a family history of that disease. Since so many more women die each year from cardiovascular disease, it is of paramount importance that women pay the same attention to their risk factors and family history for heart disease.

Although we can do nothing about the genes passed on to us by our parents, women—both with and without a family history of heart disease—can make many vital changes to modify and lower other risk factors for coronary heart disease. Obviously, early and more aggressive testing may be indicated for those with a positive family history.

## 4. THE DANGER OF DIABETES IN WOMEN

Gloria is a fifty-year-old woman who is overweight and has a sedentary lifestyle. At her annual visit to the doctor, she was surprised to hear that she had high sugar levels and qualified as a diabetic. As her doctor explained what diabetes meant to her health, she was shocked to know this condition put her, in turn at risk for heart disease.

Many women are unaware that diabetes is a significant risk factor for coronary heart disease and that this risk is greater in women as compared with men.[4] Approximately twenty-four million women have mildly elevated sugar levels (fasting blood glucose level of 100 to 125 mg/dl); this is called prediabetes, and it puts a woman at a higher risk for ultimately developing diabetes. A full eight million women have been diagnosed with diabetes (fasting blood glucose levels ≥ 126 mg/dL). In addition, 2.5 million women have significantly elevated sugar levels and have true diabetes, but they are unaware they have the disease. Ninety percent of diabetes is type 2 (adult-onset) diabetes that occurs when an organ in the body, the pancreas, produces too little of the hormone insulin and/or when the body's tissues become resistant to normal or even high levels of insulin. The body needs insulin to take the sugar from the blood into the cells. When sugar builds up in the blood instead, it can cause health problems. High blood sugar levels can lead to the development of heart disease, with damage to the blood vessels in the body and injury to other organs as well. Ten percent of people have type 1 diabetes, which is a chronic medical condition that occurs when the pancreas produces no insulin or very little. Usually, type 1 diabetes develops in children and young adults.

Several factors are associated with developing diabetes. The first is genetic: 39 percent of patients with type 2 diabetes have at least one parent with type 2 diabetes. In addition, Asians, Hispanics, and African Americans are at higher risk for developing diabetes, compared with Caucasians. In women who are pregnant, 3–5 percent will develop gestational diabetes, which is defined as glucose intolerance of variable degree, and classically deliver babies who weigh ten pounds or more at birth. Although gestational diabetes disappears shortly after childbirth, these women are at higher risk for developing primarily type 2 diabetes as they get older.[5]

Lifestyle is an important factor in the development of diabetes and interacts with the genetic predisposition for the disease. Although diabetes was once considered a disease of older people, we are seeing it more frequently in younger women, and this is likely related to the increase in obesity and physical inactivity in our society.

Diabetes affects multiple areas of the body. One of the most important is the heart because approximately 75 percent of women with diabetes will die from a heart attack or stroke.[6] It is essential that women get an early diagnosis because with control of their blood sugar levels through appropriate medications and lifestyle modifications—including regular exercise, weight management, smoking cessation, and proper nutrition—they can minimize their risk of heart disease and other potential diabetic complications. These complications can include damage to their sight, nerve damage, poor wound healing, toe or lower limb amputation, and kidney failure.

# 5. TOBACCO CAN MAKE A WOMAN'S LIFE GO UP IN SMOKE

Tobacco use in women not only ages your skin but may cost you your life! Over 50 percent of women who have angina or heart attacks are smokers. In women, even smoking only one to four cigarettes a day will double the chance that you will have a heart attack or die from one.[7] If you have other risk factors for heart disease—such as high blood pressure, being overweight, a positive family history for heart disease, or diabetes—you are at an even greater risk if you smoke. There is good news though. If you stop smoking, the increased risk for heart disease will decrease to that of a woman who has never smoked, within two to three years after you stop. It can be very, very hard to stop smoking, but the benefits are worth the trouble. Talk to your doctor about medications such as nicotine patches, nicotine nasal spray, Zyban, and Chantix as well as behavioral programs that can help you win this battle.

# 6. HYPERTENSION: THE SILENT KILLER OF WOMEN

High blood pressure is very common in women as they get older. In fact, 70 to 80 percent of women over the age of seventy years have high blood pressure. Especially in older women, high blood pressure is a very significant risk factor for developing heart disease and stroke—more so than in men of the same age. But high blood pressure is not only a risk for older women. In premenopausal women, there is a tenfold increased risk of dying from cardiovascular disease if they have high blood pressure. High blood pressure is called a "silent killer" because women often are completely unaware that they have it—they feel fine. The treatment of high blood pressure can sometimes be relatively easy, with changes in your lifestyle such as decreasing the amount of salt in your diet (take the salt shaker off the dinner table, use salt substitutes, and avoid canned and processed foods), losing weight if you are obese or overweight, decreasing the amount of alcohol you drink (women should not have more than one drink a day), and increasing your physical activity to at least thirty minutes of exercise three times per week. Dr. Caulin-Glaser and her husband started walking after dinner. It helps digestion, promotes conversation, and greatly benefits our hearts. However, some women will still need blood pressure treatment through medications. Your doctor will likely talk to you about starting a medication if the systolic pressure (the top number) is above 140 mmHg and/or the diastolic pressure (the bottom number) is above 90 mmHg, after having measured your blood pressure several times and after you've made the lifestyle changes discussed above. Many times, patients will argue with their doctor about having to take medications since they are feeling fine—it seems like an unnecessary expense. I often wish those individuals were able to see the devastating results of a stroke or heart attack in my patients who refused to take medications to control their blood pressure.

# 7. ARE WOMEN TREATED APPROPRIATELY FOR HIGH CHOLESTEROL?

*You should know your cholesterol numbers as well as you know your dress size.*

Women need to be aware that there are differences between men and women when it comes to cholesterol numbers and risk of heart disease. In addition to knowing the "bad" cholesterol, low-density lipoprotein (or LDL) level, women must also ask their doctor about another cholesterol level, the "good" cholesterol, or high-density lipoprotein (HDL). A low "good" cholesterol number is a very important risk factor for heart disease in women. Women should have a HDL cholesterol level of 50 mg/dL or greater. They should have a LDL level less than 150 mg/dl. Another number women should know is their triglyceride level (another type of fat in the blood), because triglycerides also affect the risk of getting heart disease, especially in older women. Your triglyceride levels should be less than 150 mg/dl. Every woman over age twenty should have a "fasting" cholesterol profile measured. Fasting means "nothing to eat or drink after midnight" and your lab test taken first thing in the morning. All women need to know their cholesterol numbers and have discussions with their doctor about their risk for heart disease and the potential need for treatment. Lifestyle changes can help keep cholesterol numbers in a healthy range. One change is regular aerobic exercise (aerobic means "with oxygen," and aerobic exercise is defined as any extended duration exercise of low to moderate difficulty that uses the large muscle groups of the body, such as the legs or back). Other changes include maintaining an appropriate body weight and decreasing the amount of saturated fat in your diet. Determining if you need to be treated with medications for your cholesterol requires your doctor to take into consideration multiple potential risk factors, such as your blood pressure, age, and use of tobacco, as well as cholesterol levels. Using a tool called the Framingham Risk Score (www.nhlbi.nih.gov) allows your doctor to calculate your specific risk, as a woman, for a heart event over the next ten years. Ask your doctor what your score is because, unfortunately, women are often undertreated for abnormal cholesterol levels.

## 8. OBESITY: THE GROWING RISK FACTOR FOR WOMEN OF ALL AGES

The National Health and Nutrition Examination Survey (NHANES) 2003–2004 reported that 34 percent of women between the ages of twenty to seventy are obese.[8] This represents a daunting increase from 1976 to 1980, when only 17 percent of women were obese. What is causing this epidemic of obesity? The answer is complicated because many factors have played a role, including a decrease in physical activity, increased portion sizes, fast foods, more sedentary jobs, increased use of computers/TV, and driving our cars rather than walking. Obesity is associated with an increased risk for heart disease. Obese women often have additional risk factors for heart disease, such as high blood pressure, low "good" cholesterol levels, high triglyceride levels, and high glucose or "sugar" levels—that can be an indication of prediabetes or type 2 diabetes. So how do we know if we are obese? The body mass index (BMI) is the most common way to make that determination. It is calculated from the height and weight as follows:

BMI = body weight (in kilograms) ÷ square of height (in meters)
   To calculate your own body mass index, do the following:
   1. Multiply your weight in pounds by 703.
   2. Divide by your height in inches (for example, 5 feet 4 inches = 64 inches)
   3. Divide again by your height in inches

Let's do the following example. If you were 5'4" and weighed 130 pounds, your BMI calculation would look like this:
       Step 1. $130 \times 703 = 91,390$
       Step 2. $91,390 \div 64 = 1,427.96$
       Step 3. $1,427.96 \div 64 = 22.3$
       The answer: Your BMI would be 22.2 kg/m².

Most men and women in the United States are more familiar with using pounds and inches to express their weight and height, but BMI is universally expressed in kilograms and meters. Let's review the numbers you need to remember. The goal is to have a BMI less than 25 kg/m². You are considered overweight if your BMI is between 25 and 29.9 kg/m² and obese if your BMI is greater than or equal to 30 kg/m². At any given level of BMI, the risk to your heart health is increased by having an increased amount of abdominal fat, or fat around your waist. For women, this would mean that your waist measurement is greater than 35-inches. Your doctor should measure your waist during your physical evaluations. The good news is that with weight loss you can make some important strides toward a healthy heart, such as decreasing your blood pressure, decreasing the risk of developing diabetes, improving cholesterol levels, and reducing inflammation (internal "irritation" of your body tissues). Inflammation is another risk factor for heart disease to be discussed later in this book.

If you need to lose weight, it is essential for both you and your doctor to set realistic weight-loss goals. If you try a "fad" diet and lose weight rapidly, you will likely gain it back. I ask my patients before they start a diet, "Can you see yourself eating the same way as on your diet in one year, two years, or five years from now?" I ask this question because what is important is a sustained lifestyle change, not just trying to fit into a bathing suit for an upcoming vacation! A realistic goal is to lose 5 percent of your initial weight over a six-month period. If you are able to accomplish this goal and then maintain the weight loss for three months, then set another goal of 5 percent weight loss. A quick way to determine how many calories you need each day is as follows:

# of pounds you currently weigh $\times$ 15 = the number of calories needed daily

As an example: if you weigh 130 pounds, multiply $130 \times 15$, and you get 1,950 calories; this represents the average number of calories a moderately active person will need to maintain that weight. If you are less active, you would use thirteen as the multiplication factor instead of fifteen. To lose weight, you will need to either take in fewer calories or be more active to burn calories. Remember that one pound equals thirty-five hundred calories. In the appendix of this book are some exercises to help increase your physical activity. Increasing physical activity will help burn calories and is also associated with other health benefits such as these:

- Helps you have more energy, enhancing daily activity
- Helps control weight
- Lowers high blood pressure
- Lowers high cholesterol
- Reduces the risk of diabetes
- Reduces the risk of heart disease
- Reduces the risk of colon and breast cancer
- Improves control of preexisting heart risk factors
- Promotes psychological well-being
- Helps maintain healthy bones, muscles, and joints
- Reduces the risk of osteoporosis
- Reduces musculoskeletal injuries
- Improves self-esteem

Small dietary modifications can make a big difference in your weight. If you can eliminate one can of soda (approximately 250 calories) from your diet each day, you will lose approximately one pound every two weeks.

Write down everything you put into your mouth (food and drink) for one week. Sit down and review the list at the end of the week and choose one item from each day that you can easily go without. We have included some help for you when it comes to managing your weight with samples of how to create 1,400-, 1,800-, and 2,200-calorie diets, a great snack list, and how to choose the "better" bad when eating at fast-food places.

**Daily Needs:**

| | | |
|---|---|---|
| Calories: 1400 | Protein: 6 ounces | |
| Carb. Grams: 165 | Fats: 3-4 servings | |
| Carb.# Choices: 11 | | |

**Daily Needs:**

| | | |
|---|---|---|
| Calories: 1800 | Protein: 8 ounces | |
| Carb. Grams: 215 | Fats: 3-4 servings | |
| Carb. # Choices: 14 | | |

**Daily Needs:**

| | | |
|---|---|---|
| Calories: 2000 | Protein: 9 ounces | |
| Carb. Grams: 225 | Fats: 4-5 servings | |
| Carb. # Choices: 15 | | |

| Meals/Snacks | CARBOHYDRATES<br>Starch<br>Fruite<br>Milk/Yogurt | PROTEIN<br>Meats<br>Eggs<br>Cheese/Nuts/Peanut Butter | FATS<br>Oils<br>Margarine<br>Salad Dressing | VEGETABLES<br>Onions<br>Spinach<br>Green Beans<br>FREE |
|---|---|---|---|---|
| Breakfast | Grams ___ Calories ___ | Calories ___ | Servings ___ | |
| Lunch | Grams ___ Calories ___ | Calories ___ | Servings ___ | |
| Dinner | Grams ___ Calories ___ | Calories ___ | Servings ___ | |

## CARBOHYDRATES

| Starch | Fruit |
|---|---|
| Choose whole grain breads and cereals (bran, wheat, oats) | Choose more fresh fruits than juices. They have more fiber. |
| • Use beans as an excellent source of fiber<br>• Try whole wheat pasta and brown rice<br>• Low-fat snack foods include pretzels, low-fat wheat crackers, and air popped popcorn | • Eat a good variety of fresh fruits<br>• Select "lite" canned fruits or fruits canned in their own juices rather than in syrup |
| Milk/Yogurt | Sweets |
| Choose low fat milks: skim or 1% | Choose sweets less often, they are high in fat and sugar |
| • Choose "lite" or plain low-fat yogurt<br>• Try plain low-fat soy milk for variety | • When choosing sweets, include them in your carbohydrate budget, not in addition to it |

## VEGETABLES

• Choose mainly fresh or frozen vegetables without added sauces, fats, or salt
• Include three or more servings of vegetables in your day

## MEATS AND OTHERS

Meats and Others

- Choose fish and poultry more often than beef or pork
- Trim all visible fat from meat
- Bake, grill, roast, boil, and broil instead of frying or using heavy sauces or gravies

## FATS

Fats

- Eat fewer fats
- Monounsaturated fats such as those in nuts, olive and canola oil, and avocado are healthier choices
- Eat less saturated fat by reducing use of cheese, bacon, butter, and sweets

## DINING OUT
## The Fast Food Challenge

| An "Unhappy" Meal | Cals | Fat | Carb | A "Happy" Meal Choice | Cals | Fat | Carb |
|---|---|---|---|---|---|---|---|
| **Wendy's** | | | | **Wendy's** | | | |
| Spicy Chicken Sandwich | 410 | 14 | 43 | Grilled Chicken Sandwich | 300 | 7 | 36 |
| Biggie Fries | 470 | 23 | 61 | Side Salad w/lowfat Ranch dressing | 180 | 14 | 9 |
| Pepsi (11 oz..) | 130 | 0 | 36 | Diet Pepsi | 0 | 0 | 0 |
| Total: | 1010 | 37 | 140 | Total | 480 | 21 | 45 |
| **Subway** | | | | **Subway** | | | |
| 6" meatball sub | 501 | 25 | 45 | Subway Club | 294 | 5 | 40 |
| 1 bag potato chips | 230 | 15 | 23 | 1 bag baked potato chips | 130 | 15 | 26 |
| Diet Coke | 0 | 0 | 0 | Ice Water | 0 | 0 | 0 |
| Total: | 731 | 40 | 69 | Total: | 424 | 65 | 66 |
| **KFC** | | | | **KFC** | | | |
| Original recipe breast | 400 | 24 | 16 | Tender roast w/o skin | 170 | 4.5 | 1 |
| Biscuit | 180 | 10 | 20 | Corn on cob | 150 | 2 | 35 |
| Baked beans | 190 | 3 | 33 | Mashed potatoes/gravy | 120 | 6 | 17 |
| Coleslaw | 232 | 14 | 26 | Total: | 440 | 13 | 53 |
| Total: | 1002 | 51 | 95 | | | | |
| **Pizza Hut** | | | | **Pizza Hut** | | | |
| Meat Lover's pan pizza 3 slices | 1290 | 63 | 135 | Veggie Lover's Thin & Crispy 3 slices | 660 | 24 | 90 |
| **McDonald's** | | | | **McDonald's** | | | |
| Sausage biscuit w/egg | 505 | 33 | 33 | Egg McMuffin | 280 | 11 | 28 |
| Hashbrown | 130 | 7 | 15 | Small apple or small milk | 60 | 0 | 15 |
| Orange juice (5oz.) | 80 | 0 | 20 | Total: | 340 | 11 | 43 |
| Total: | 715 | 40 | 68 | | | | |
| **Taco Bell** | | | | **Taco Bell** | | | |
| Nachos supreme | 440 | 24 | 44 | Chicken soft taco | 190 | 7 | 19 |
| Beef burrito | 430 | 18 | 50 | Mexican rice | 190 | 9 | 23 |
| Total: | 880 | 42 | 94 | Total: | 380 | 16 | 42 |
| **Boston Market** | | | | **Boston Market** | | | |
| dark meat chicken | 320 | 21 | 2 | white meat chicken | 280 | 12 | 2 |
| Macarroni & cheese | 280 | 11 | 32 | New potatoes | 130 | 3 | 25 |
| Creamed spinach | 260 | 20 | 11 | Zucchini marinara | 60 | 3 | 7 |
| Cornbread | 200 | 6 | 33 | Cornbread | 100 | 3 | 16 |
| Total: | 1060 | 58 | 78 | Total: | 570 | 21 | 50 |
| **Chinese** | | | | **Chinese** | | | |
| Egg roll | 250 | 15 | 18 | Egg drop soup (1 C) | 50 | 3 | 2 |
| Sweet & sour pork | 950 | 50 | 92 | Chicken & snow peas | 200 | 17 | 7 |
| Fried rice (1C) | 370 | 12 | 48 | Steamed rice (1 C) | 120 | 0 | 50 |
| Total: | 1145 | 55 | 158 | Total | 370 | 20 | 59 |

# 9. IS YOUR DIET A HEART HEALTH HAZARD?

Katie was very upset when she arrived for her annual physical with her doctor. She went on a new diet that had been on all the TV shows and magazines. She lost fifteen pounds in only two weeks! The bad news was she regained twenty pounds over the next three months. What happened to Katie? She went on a diet that was not sustainable. Every woman needs to ask and answer the following question before starting a diet: will I be eating this way in five years? If not, then she has not chosen a change in lifestyle but only a temporary measure.

I will review recommendations for a scientifically evidence-based diet that is based on the results of many stuidies.

The most important message to women regarding their diet is moderation—moderation in types of food, quantity, and portion size. Here are some basics to include in any nutrition plan: vegetables, fruits, whole grains, broiled or baked chicken, and fish, while limiting red meat. Fiber is a key component of any diet and is associated with a decreased risk of heart disease. Fiber can be incorporated into the diet with cereals, vegetables, and fruits.

Try this technique the next time you sit down to eat. Look at your dinner plate, and if it is full of food that is all one color—beige—you need to change your diet. The dinner plate needs to be colorful. Vegetables and fruits add color to your plate, and you should aim for as much color as possible! A good rule is to avoid "white" foods, as in white bread, white rice, white potatoes, and white pasta. These foods are high in carbohydrates, are rapidly absorbed, are high in calories, and can cause increases in triglyceride levels (a type of bad cholesterol). Trans-fatty acids should be avoided as well. Examples include stick margarine, fried foods, and bakery items (cakes, cookies, donuts). Eating trans-fatty acids will

result in higher "bad" cholesterol levels and lower "good" cholesterol levels and therefore will increase your risk of heart disease.
Saturated fatty acids are also to be avoided. The most common
sources are dairy products such as milk (use skim milk instead), ice
cream (try low-fat yogurt or ice milk), cheese (choose low-fat
cheese), and meat. Some fats that may properly be included in the
diet are called monounsaturated fatty acids. These are frequently
found in olive and canola oil, but remember—moderation!

Remember to allow yourself an indulgence every now and then.
However, never let one indulgence become an excuse for giving up
on your smart-eating plan. One overindulgence should be the
exception rather than the rule. The key to success is that you eat
portion-controlled healthy foods most of the time.

# CHAPTER 5

# HOW DO YOU KNOW IF YOU HAVE A HEART PROBLEM?

Eileen is a sixty-year-old woman with a history of high blood pressure, an elevated triglyceride level, and a low HDL-C level. She went to the doctor with complaints of shoulder/upper-back discomfort and shortness of breath when she was walking her dog. Her doctor told her not to worry—she likely had arthritis and needed to lose some weight. The symptoms persisted, increasing in frequency and intensity, until finally Eileen went to the emergency room to be evaluated. The triage nurse told her to take a seat and wait: her complaints were not urgent enough to be seen immediately. Two hours later, when Eileen was finally examined and an ECG was performed, she was told she had had a heart attack.

## 1. ARE A WOMAN'S SYMPTOMS DIFFERENT FROM A MAN'S?

The answer is yes. Women feel angina and heart attack pain differently from men. Although women will most frequently feel chest pain or discomfort, they are more likely than men to have other symptoms such as shortness of breath, upper-abdominal pain/discomfort, nausea and/or vomiting, upper-back/upper-arm/shoulder discomfort, and jaw pain. It is important to recognize new recurrent symptoms and talk to your doctor about them. If you feel you are not being taken seriously, you should seek a second opinion! Unfortunately, women who go to the emergency department with new onset chest pain or discomfort are approached and diagnosed less aggressively than men. Women in the ER are more likely to receive medications "to calm their nerves" instead of appropriately aggressive evaluation and treatment!

## 2. KNOW THE SYMPTOMS

The symptoms of a heart attack vary from person to person, but those listed below are frequently described by patients. If you think you may be having a heart attack, call 911—heart muscle can be dying if you delay! Treatment can be initiated by the emergency medical technicians (EMTs), who, on the way to the hospital, are in contact with the emergency room doctors. The EMTs can also treat complications that can occur with heart attacks, such as abnormal and/or irregular heart rhythms. The following are symptoms of a heart attack:

- Discomfort in the chest is often described as a pain, fullness, burning, tightness, or squeezing sensation that usually lasts for more than five minutes. The discomfort can be constant or recurring.
- Discomfort or pain in the arms, back, neck/throat, jaw, or upper abdomen
- Shortness of breath
- Profuse sweating, nausea, or lightheadedness
- Extreme fatigue despite adequate sleep

## 3. WHAT ARE THE RISK FACTORS FOR WOMEN?

Generally, women are approximately ten years older than men when they have their first heart attack and more likely to have risk factors such as diabetes, high blood pressure, and abnormal cholesterol levels, as noted earlier. Another less common cause of damage to the heart muscle, in the absence of coronary artery disease, is stress-induced cardiomyopathy, also called "broken heart" syndrome.[1] As described earlier, it usually is precipitated by intense mental stress and occurs most frequently in postmenopausal women. Despite an often complicated hospital course, most women recover completely from broken heart syndrome within one to four weeks.

Risk factors for heart disease, which can differ between men and women, should be reviewed during all annual physical evaluations with your primary care doctor. Review and discuss the risk factors below:

- History of heart disease
- Age greater than fifty-five
- Abnormal cholesterol levels: high LDL (bad cholesterol), low HDL (good cholesterol), and high triglyceride levels
- Family history of heart disease (father or brother younger than fifty-five and/or a mother or sister younger than sixty-five when diagnosed with heart disease)
- Diabetes
- Smoking
- High blood pressure
- Obesity
- Physical inactivity
- Peripheral vascular disease (blockages to blood flow in the legs and arms)

# 4. TAKE ACTION AGAINST HEART DISEASE

The American Heart Association and the American College of Cardiology have published guidelines for the prevention of heart disease in women.[2] Below are significant actions all women can take to decrease their risk:

- Exercise at least three times per week. Try for most of the other days as well.
- Increase your daily activity in addition to exercise. Listed below are a few ways to add steps to your day:
  - ♥ Take the stairs whenever possible
  - ♥ Park farther from the store
  - ♥ Walk while on the phone
  - ♥ Walk around while watching TV
  - ♥ Try never to sit longer than one hour
  - ♥ Walk one lap around the mall before you shop
- Do not smoke; if you do smoke, use both medications and behavioral programs to help you stop.
- Eat a healthy diet low in saturated and trans-fats and rich in fruits, vegetables, and fish.
- Manage your weight; know your body mass index.
- Know all of your cholesterol numbers and if necessary take appropriate medications to reach a healthy goal. The total cholesterol level should be less than 200 mg/dL, with an HDL (good) cholesterol level greater than 50 mg/dL and a triglyceride level less than 150 mg/dL. The ideal LDL (bad) cholesterol level is determined by your risk factors for heart disease. A good level for you may not be the same as for your best friend. You need to discuss your cholesterol results with your doctor.
- Know your blood pressure. The goal is less than or equal to

120/80 mm/Hg. If necessary, make lifestyle changes and take appropriate medications to reach that goal.

- Know your fasting blood glucose level. The ideal goal is a fasting blood glucose of less than or equal to 100 mg/dL. If you are diabetic, work with your doctor on close management of glucose, blood pressure, and cholesterol levels.

## 5. CARDIAC REHABILITATION

Cardiac rehabilitation is an important treatment after a heart attack, the placement of a stent, valve surgery, or coronary bypass surgery. Comprehensive programs have been developed to: provide exercise training, patient-directed educational programs, lifestyle modifications for cardiac risk factor reduction, and psychological support in the secondary prevention (prevention of future cardiac events after a heart attack) of coronary heart disease. Participation in these programs has been shown to be associated with a 31 percent decrease in cardiovascular mortality and a 27 percent decrease in total mortality.[3] Unfortunately, very few women are referred to these programs after a cardiac event, and the participation rates have been reported as low as 10 percent for women.[4] Cardiac rehabilitation should be an integral part of secondary prevention for all patients, including women, who have had coronary events. Indeed, the American Heart Association and the American College of Cardiology promote a multifaceted approach in these patients that includes cardiac rehabilitation.[5]

To summarize, no woman is completely free from the risk of developing heart disease. Be aware of how cardiac symptoms can manifest in a woman. Even if you don't have symptoms, you should know your risk factors. Heart disease develops over time and can start at a young age. No matter what your age, practice good habits now so you can be healthy and productive later. If you have been diagnosed with heart disease, participate in cardiac rehabilitation, as the benefits are significant both in terms of heart health and quality of life.

# Chapter 6

# THE HEART OF THE MATTER ON HORMONE THERAPY AND ORAL CONTRACEPTION

Patti is a fifty-one-year-old postmenopausal woman with high cholesterol, whose mother died of a heart attack at the age of sixty-one. Patti's doctor started her on hormone replacement therapy three years ago to help prevent the development of heart dis-ease. Now Patti has heard on the news that there are risks of heart attacks and strokes with hormone replacement, and she is concerned about what to do. Should she just stop the medication? Is she now at higher risk for heart disease?

## 1. HORMONE THERAPY:

The woman described in the case above represents the great many women today who have expressed concerns about hormone therapy (HT). Using HT has become one of the most important and difficult judgments for women and their physicians to make in this decade.

Here we will help explain the changes that occur during menopause, how menopause and HT affect your risk for developing heart disease, how to make sense of the scientific studies, and how to make an informed decision with your doctor about HT.

Every health decision must be made with a clear understanding of the pertinent issues, weighing both the consequent risks as well as the benefits. Not electing to take HT quite simply eliminates any risk but also excludes any benefits.

## What Is Menopause?

Menopause is a *natural* event and a phase of woman's life in which she will spend over a third of her years. In simple terms, menopause means a woman has had her last menstrual cycle. To be considered post-menopausal, a woman must have not menstruated for twelve months.

Menopause begins when the sex hormones—estrogens, progesterone, and testosterone—produced by your ovaries fall to very low levels, and the menstrual periods regulated by these hormones stop. The levels of estrogen fall to almost a tenth of those found in pre-menopausal women, and the progesterone levels become nearly undetectable. A small amount of estrogen is still produced by the adrenal glands and by fat tissue but no longer by the ovaries.

> **FACT:** **A woman's normal sex hormones are estrogen, progesterone, and testosterone. Production of these hormones declines with menopause.**

The menopausal process involves a gradual decline in hormone production, occuring over several years during a period termed perimenopause. Peri is a Greek word for "near" or "about." During perimenopause, a woman will still experience her menstrual cycle, but it may become irregular, often skipping a month. Ovulation becomes less predictable, and fertility rates become significantly lower. A blood test for the follicle stimulating hormone (FSH) level is useful in confirming that you are in menopause. Most commonly, menopause, happens naturally between the ages of forty-five and fifty-five, although it can occur as early as thirty-five or as late as fifty-nine. Menopause also can be advanced very rapidly via a surgical intervention: a young woman may have a pelvic operation and her ovaries removed for a variety of gynecologic indications.

Many physical and emotional changes can be associated with this transition. The most frequent are:

> Hot flashes
> Sleep problems
> Sweating
> Vaginal dryness
> Weight gain
> Hair loss
> Abnormal vaginal bleeding pattern
> Decrease in sex drive
> Urinary incontinence
> Osteoporosis

## What Is Hormone Therapy?

Hormone therapy compensates for the loss of sex hormones that occurs with menopause. Hormone therapy is a medically prescribed formulation of either estrogen therapy (ET) alone or in combination with a second hormone called progestin, a synthetic form of progesterone (HT). Estrogen is a female hormone that affects many organs.

> Bones
> Blood vessels
> Brain
> Urogenital
> Breast
> Adipose (fat) tissue

If you and your doctor have decided you need hormone therapy, both estrogen and progestin therapy are necessary for women who have a uterus. Estrogen alone stimulates the lining of the uterus. Natural progesterone levels fall in the second half of a woman's menstrual cycle, triggering the shedding of the estrogen-stimulated uterine lining if pregnancy has not occurred. Unopposed estrogen for long periods increases the risk of endometrial cancer (cancer of the lining of the uterus).

To eliminate the infrequent but potentially grave risk of uterine cancer, only postmenopausal women without a uterus would be treated with estrogen-only therapy. Estrogen therapy doubles the level of estrogen found in a postmenopausal woman but never reaches that of a premenopausal woman. A variety of different estrogen preparations are used for the symptoms associated with menopause. The most common are listed below along with the available progesterone preparations.

| Oral Estrogen | Estradiol Patches | Estrogen Gel/Patch/ Vaginal Ring |
|---|---|---|
| Estrace | Alora | Estrogel |
| Gynodiol | Climara | Estrasorb |
| Menest | Esclim | Femring |
| Ogen | Estraderm | |
| Ortho-est | Vivelle | |
| Premarin | | |
| Cenestin | | |
| Enjuvia | | |

**Progesterone**

Provera-pill

Cycrin-pill

Micronized (natural progesterone)-pill

**HEALTH TIP:** **You should not take estrogen alone for hormone replacement, unless your uterus has already been removed. Estrogen alone promotes endometrial cancer of the uterus.**

## Why Use Hormone Therapy?

Traditionally, HT has been used short term to relieve the symptoms of menopause as previously described on page 105. In addition, over the years, the role of HT has been expanded to include its longer-term use—to prevent the development of chronic diseases commonly seen in menopausal women, such as osteoporosis and heart disease. Recent clinical trials have given us more information about the role of HT for the prevention and/or treatment of chronic disease. The overall recommendation is that HT is *not* appropriate for the prevention of chronic diseases such as osteoporosis and heart disease. (We will review the important hormone studies on which this conclusion is based later in this chapter.)

**HEALTH TIP: Newer studies show that hormone replacement therapy is not appropriate for long-term use for the prevention of chronic diseases, such as osteoporosis and heart disease.**

It is important to remember that menopause is *not* a disease. Women generally live twenty to forty years after the onset of menopause and need to be assertive about their heart and general health.

## Will You Get Heart Disease after Menopause?

Heart disease increases in both men and women with advancing age. By the age of fifty, 50 percent of male deaths are due to heart disease, as compared with only 10 percent at the age of twenty.[1] In general, women have a ten-year lag in the development of heart disease. By the age of sixty, 50 percent of female deaths are from heart disease.[2]

> **FACT:** **Heart disease lags by about ten years in women as opposed to men. In men, by age fifty, half of deaths are due to heart disease. In women, this landmark is not reached until sixty years of age.**

For many years, scientists believed that the delayed development of heart disease in women was due to the beneficial effects of naturally produced estrogen, including improved cholesterol levels, decreased levels of blood-clotting proteins, direct protection of the blood vessel walls, antioxidant effects to prevent cholesterol buildup in the blood vessels, and increased production of nitric oxide, a substance that relaxes the blood vessels (not nitrous oxide used by the dentist!).

After menopause, the risk of developing heart disease does increase in women. This *does not* mean that all women will develop heart disease after menopause, but it does mean that a woman needs to be aware that cardiovascular disease is the number-one killer of women in the United States, claiming over 460,000 women every year.[3]

In the next several pages, we will review the results of some important studies looking at the impact of hormone therapy on your risk of developing heart disease.

# Does Hormone Therapy Increase or Decrease the Risk of Heart Disease?

To answer this question, we need to understand the scientific studies that have been done looking at HT and heart disease and how they were conducted. In order to be valid, a scientific study must account for all the possible factors that may influence the single effect being measured. For example, say we set up a study to see if HT decreases heart disease. The women in Group 1 of our study receive a placebo (pill that has no effect) and, just by chance, happen to smoke cigarettes; the women in Group 2 receive HT but also, just by chance, do not smoke cigarettes. If, when we look at these women in one year, we find more heart disease in Group 1, it may be the result of the negative health effect of cigarette smoking as opposed to the benefit of HT given to Group 2. Many factors besides estrogen may contribute to the development of heart disease in women.

Research and clinical studies on women's health are vital. Until the past decade, women were frequently not included in clinical studies of heart disease. When they were, the information was analyzed as a group that included *both* men and women, so the results for women were not looked at separately. Some major questions regarding women's heart disease are now being asked and answered by the medical community. The National Institutes of Health and other agencies have recently promoted and even mandated specific investigations on heart disease and its treatment in women. Now let's look at the actual studies.

## *Observational Studies*

Over thirty observational studies have been published examining the effect of HT on heart disease in women. The majority suggested that there was an approximately 50 percent decrease in the risk of heart disease with the use of HT.[4]

One of the most important observational studies that indicated the benefits to the heart from estrogen was the Nurses' Health Study. Investigators followed 122,000 nurses between the ages of thirty and fifty-five. The fifteen-year follow-up, reported in 1994, showed significantly fewer heart attacks (a 40 percent decrease) in women taking estrogen therapy compared to women not taking estrogen. Nevertheless, a concern in this study was an increase in stroke and breast cancer in women on estrogen therapy.

It is important to understand the limitations of this type of study. An observational study involves selecting a group of women and comparing them with another group of women. The investigators do not interfere with the subjects' medications or lifestyles. For estrogen studies, women taking the hormone were compared with women not taking the medication. The scientists observed only what happened to these women over time.

The heart benefit found in the estrogen group may have been related to socioeconomic status or to healthier lifestyles, not to the estrogen replacement. They may have exercised regularly, maintained a healthy weight, followed a low-fat diet, not smoked, and monitored their blood pressure and cholesterol levels better, compared with the women not taking HT. In addition, women on HT may have had more frequent and regular physician visits because they were taking a prescribed medication. These visits could have promoted better prevention, as well as diagnosis and treatment, of heart disease.

### Postmenopausal Estrogen/Progestin Interventions Trial (PEPI)

This was a National Institutes of Health–supported study to look at the effect of HT on cardiac risk factors in *healthy postmenopausal* women. The PEPI trial was a prospective, randomized, double-blind, placebo-controlled study.[5]

Again, it is important to understand how the study was designed. This is an example of a very well-designed clinical test. In a double-blind study, women are asked to volunteer and be randomly assigned to take one of four hormone therapies or a placebo. Random assignment is like flipping a coin to decide who goes first in a game. This is the only way that the investigators can be fairly sure that other factors, such as exercise habits, smoking, diet, and the like, will not affect the study, because there is an equal chance of a woman with specific habits being assigned to each arm of the study. As the other part of the double-blind study, the scientists are not told what medication each group is taking so that their own bias (their feelings on how the study results should look) does not interfere with interpreting the study results.

The study enrolled 875 postmenopausal women who took one of four types of hormone replacement: daily estrogen alone, daily estrogen with progestin (a synthetic progesterone), daily estrogen with progestin twelve days of the month, daily estrogen with a natural progesterone, or placebo (no active hormone). The results compared with the placebo (pill that had no effect ) group were as follows:

a. All four types of hormone replacements increased HDL-C (the good cholesterol) levels. The most impressive increases were with estrogen alone or estrogen with progesterone. (Good.)

b. All four types of hormone replacements decreased LDL-C (the bad cholesterol) levels. This was a good effect. (Good.)

c. Fibrinogen, a substance that causes clots to form in the blood and is associated with increased risk of heart attacks, was decreased with all four types of hormone replacement. (Good.)

d. None of the hormone replacement therapies caused an increase in weight, blood pressure, or insulin levels. (Neutral.)

e. All four of the hormone therapies increased the blood triglyceride levels. (Bad.)

f. All hormone replacement therapies increased bone density, which is a risk factor for the development of osteoporosis. (Good.)

g. Estrogen-only therapy caused abnormal cell growth (hyperplasia) in the lining of the uterus. (Bad.) Women who had a hysterectomy did not have this risk because the uterus had been removed.

### *Heart and Estrogen/Progestin Replacement Study I and II Trial (HERS)*

This was a randomized, double-blind, placebo-controlled study of daily estrogen and progestin (synthetic progesterone) therapy or placebo in postmenopausal women who had documented coronary artery disease (heart attack).[6] This study was designed to see if it helped prevent the progression of established heart disease. HERS I and II Trials differed from the PEPI Trial because all the women *already had heart disease*; the women in the PEPI Trial were healthy. In addition, only one type of HT and pattern of administration were used in this study. The HERS I Trial was extended (HERS II) so that 2,321 women were followed for 6.8 years.[7] The HERS Trial demonstrated the following:

a. A *significantly increased risk* of a heart attack in the *first* year of starting HT. (Bad.)

b. A small but *not significantly decreased* risk of heart disease compared with placebo at the completion of the study, 6.8 years (366 vs. 368 heart attacks annually per 10,000 women).

(Neutral.) (Note that in medical studies, the term *not statistically significant* means that the observed effect may well just be due to chance. This vernacular implies that the effect in question has failed to be demonstrated conclusively.)

c. A small but *not significantly increased* risk of stroke compared with the placebo at the completion of the study (212 vs. 195 events annually per 10,000 women). (Neutral.)

d. A *significant increase* in the risk of blood clot compared with the placebo at the completion of the study (59 vs. 28 events annually per 10,000 women). (Bad.)

e. A *significant increase* in incidence of biliary tract surgery (gallbladder) compared with the placebo at the completion of the study (191 vs. 129 events annually per 10,000 women). (Bad.)

f. A small but *not significantly decreased* risk of colon cancer compared with the placebo at the completion of the study (25 vs. 31 events annually per 10,000 women). (Neutral.)

g. A small but *not significantly increased* risk of breast cancer compared with the placebo at the completion of the study (59 vs. 47 events annually per 10,000 women). (Neutral.)

h. A small but *not significantly increased* risk of osteoporotic fracture compared with the placebo (297 vs. 284 events annually per 10,000 women). (Neutral.)

### The Women's Health Initiative (WHI)

This fifteen-year study on disease prevention in women focused specifically on heart disease, breast cancer, colorectal cancer, and osteoporosis.[8] Osteoporosis is a thinning of the bones that can result in an increased risk for bone fractures. The study began in 1991 and in involved over 161,000 *healthy postmenopausal* women. One arm of the study involved postmenopausal women who still had a uterus and took both estrogen and progestin or a placebo. These women were followed to see if the hormone therapy would help prevent heart disease and hip fracture, while they were monitored for the risks of blood clots, breast cancer, and endometrial (lining of the uterus) cancer. After 5.2 years, this part of the WHI was stopped by the safety committee because the risks of taking estrogen and progestin were greater than the risks associated with not taking the medication, as shown below:

   a. A *significantly increased* risk of heart disease compared with the placebo (37 vs. 30 events annually per 10,000 women). (Bad.)

   b. A *significantly increased* risk of stroke compared with the placebo (29 vs. 21 events annually per 10,000 women). (Bad.)

   c. A *significant increase* in the risk of blood clots compared with the placebo (34 vs. 16 events annually per 10,000 women). (Bad.)

   d. A *significantly decreased* risk of colon cancer compared with the placebo (10 vs. 16 events annually per 10,000 women). (Good.)

   e. A small but *not significantly increased* risk of breast cancer compared with the placebo (38 vs. 30 events annually per 10,000 women). (Neutral.)

   f. A *significantly decreased* risk of osteoporotic fracture compared with the placebo (146 vs. 191 events annually per 10,000 women). (Good.)

   g. No increased risk of death from breast cancer or any other cause of death.

In table 6.1, the statistically significant results of the major prospective trials of hormone therapy studies will be summarized. These are all prospective, randomized, double-blind, placebo-controlled studies. A check mark indicates a good result, and an X indicates a bad result. "CAD" refers to coronary artery disease. Note the huge number of women in the WHI study.

**Table 6.1. Statistically significant findings of major prospective trials of hormone therapy.**

| Name/ Date | # women | Study Population | Findings | | |
|---|---|---|---|---|---|
| | | | Heart | Bone | Other |
| PEPI/ 1997 | 875 | Healthy, post-menopausal | √⇑HDL-C (good cholesterol) √⇓LDL-C (bad cholesterol) √⇓fibrogen (clotting) X⇑tri-glycerides (fats in blood) | √⇑ bone density | X endome-trial hyper-trophy (bad over-growth of lining of uterus) |
| HERS I & II 2001 2002 | 2321 | Post-menopausal women with CAD (heart attack) | X⇑risk heart attack X⇑ blood clots | | X⇑gall bladder surgery |
| WHI/ 2002 | 161,000 | Healthy post-menopausal women | X⇑ heart disease X⇑ stroke X⇑ blood clots | √⇓ osteo-porosis | √⇓ colon cancer |

Okay, we have reviewed the studies—now what does this information mean for you and your decision about the use of HT? The American Heart Association, the American College of Obstetrics and Gynecology, and the US Preventive Services Task Force have recommended a similar approach to this issue for both women and physicians to use as guidelines.

## Clinical Recommendations

- The main reason for being on hormone replacement should be to relieve symptoms of menopause such as hot flashes and vaginal dryness.
- Use progesterone with estrogen only if you have a uterus.
- *Do not* use estrogen and progesterone for the prevention of heart disease.
- Consider other therapies for preventing osteoporosis.

Other available medications have proven beneficial for women at risk or with heart disease, especially for cholesterol management. The use of the medications, called statins, has been shown to decrease the risk of developing heart disease as well as death from heart disease in women. This benefit has never been shown in any study of hormone replacement.

Because there are risks with using estrogen and progesterone, *seriously* consider other therapies for the treatment of osteoporosis. Exercise and calcium supplements are important ways you can help yourself. Most important, talk to your doctor about your individual risks and benefits and whether other medications may be right for you.

Hormone therapy medications confer an increased risk of breast cancer. So if you do use HT, use estrogen and progesterone for the shortest time possible. Based on the studies we have, most of the risks of breast cancer accrue with long-term use.

If you do choose HT, always use the lowest doses of hormone possible.

Above all: *know your risks for taking hormone replacements before starting these medications and make an informed decision!*

**REMEMBER**: **Do not use HT to prevent heart disease. Other nonhormonal medications (statins) are safer and more effective.**

**REMEMBER**: **Consider exercise and calcium supplementation, <u>rather</u> than HT, for the prevention of osteoporosis.**

*The evolving nature of medicine's understanding.* There is still much that is unknown about the complicated questions of if, when, and how to use hormone therapy. The information we have just reviewed is based primarily on one type of hormone therapy—conjugated equine estrogen with progestin (commonly called Premarin and Provera). More research is needed to address the risks and benefits of different types of estrogen and progesterone, dosing schedules, and routes of administration.

## Are You Confused by the Media Reports?

Television, newspapers, radio, and the Internet all have a tremendous impact on our understanding of medical studies. Theirs is a very important role but it needs to be put into perspective. The primary function of the media should not be to substitute for your healthcare providers. Media medical reporting needs to be fair and balanced, covering all aspects of a medical issue, not just one or two recent studies that may be very controversial, poorly done, or sensational. The author and the source of the publication should be stated in any media report. Many medical experts may offer conflicting opinions about a new study, which can often make it confusing for the audience to comprehend the health implications. Understanding the type of scientific study is very crucial to deciding how accurate and relevant the information may be to your actual health. The ability to read critically and analyze scientific reports *requires* professional medical input, not just that of a favorite newscaster. It is critical to your health that you not change medications before discussing all relevant health information you may have read, heard, or seen with your physician. Your physician can put reports of any specific single study from the media into perspective vis-à-vis the overall body of knowledge.

## Is There a Role for Selective Estrogen Receptor Modulators (SERMs)?

Designed to prevent osteoporosis, these medications act by blocking estrogen receptors. Raloxifene is an example of a SERM. This drug has been studied in the Multiple Outcomes of Raloxifene Evaluation (MORE) trial, a randomized, double-blind, placebo-controlled trial.[8] The study showed that Raloxifene was associated with a decrease in spine fracture in postmenopausal women with osteoporosis. In reanalyzing the data for heart disease protection, some researchers believe that there is a decrease in heart attacks in women taking this medication. It is important to be cautious when a study is "reanalyzed." The study was not originally set up to answer the question about heart disease; therefore, other confounding factors may be contributing to the findings. An ongoing trial—Raloxifene Use for the Heart (RUTH)—will help determine if SERMs are truly helpful for heart disease prevention. There is as of yet no convincing information that this type of medication is cardio-protective.

## 2. ORAL CONTRACEPTION:

Lisa is a thirty-five year-old woman with two children. She maintains her weight, exercises three times a week, follows a low-fat diet, and smokes cigarettes. She tells her doctor that she had diabetes with her last pregnancy, but it resolved itself after the baby was born. Lisa would like to begin using oral contraception and has come to her doctor for advice.

The overall likelihood of a healthy young woman having a heart attack is low. It is essential, however, to know that the risk of a heart attack and blood clots is increased in young women who use oral contraceptives (OC). This includes the high-dose OC as well as second-generation OCs. Cardiac risk factors need to be considered when evaluating potential use of OC.

1. Smoking. Any woman who smokes should make quitting her number-one priority. This is especially the case if you are on or are considering the use of OC. Cigarette smoking increases the risk of heart disease as well as blood-clot formation. This risk increases with the age of the woman, especially after thirty-five. If a woman is to take OC, she needs to stop smoking or find another form of birth control.

2. Blood pressure. Any woman with high blood pressure needs to consider alternative methods of birth control. Blood pressure increases with the use of OC and therefore must be monitored on a regular basis while using this medication.

3. Diabetes. The regulation of glucose (blood sugar) can be dramatically affected by OC. If you have diabetes or are at risk for developing diabetes, you need to monitor your blood-glucose levels on a regular basis. This is of paramount

significance because diabetes is one of the most important risk factors for heart disease in women.

4. Stroke. Your physician, prior to starting OC, should review any preexisting health conditions you may have. This is particularly critical regarding any history you may have of strokes or ministrokes. The use of OC is associated with more frequent blood-clot formation and can increase the risk of another stroke. If you have had a stroke, you should use an alternative form of contraception.

5. Physician advice. All past medical or surgical histories need to be discussed in an open and frank manner with your doctor. This includes history of blood clots, migraines, heart defects you may have had when you were a child, and, most importantly, *any* drug (prescribed or illicit), herbal product, health food product, vitamin supplement, or over-the-counter medication you use.

**REMEMBER: Approach oral contraceptive therapy with caution if you smoke, have high blood pressure, have diabetes, or have a history of stroke or ministroke.**

It is our hope that much of the confusion and many of the questions you have had about HT and OC have been addressed and clarified. The issues concerning the use of hormone replacement are complicated, and so much more research will have to be done before we have all the answers. Fortunately, some well-designed studies have given us guidance in regard to one type of hormone replacement therapy, estrogen and progestin, and we can expect further information over the next few years from the WHI.

The most important messages we can give you:

**(1) Hormone therapy is not cardio-protective.**

**(2) Hormone therapy carries cardiac and noncardiac risks.**

**(3) Oral contraceptives confer cardiac risk in patients with other risk factors.**

Above all, be sure to discuss any and all information about hormone replacement and OC with your physician before making a decision. Please avoid the urge to view magazines, news reports, and Internet sites as "expert" or conclusive information in this or any other medical field.

# 7

# MEDICATIONS TO TREAT
# HEART DISEASE

Medications, herbal or natural supplements, and vitamins can all have side effects, interactions, or reasons why they should not be taken. Every woman — especially if she is considering becoming pregnant or is pregnant—should talk to her physician about any prescribed or over-the-counter substance she is taking. The information below is a brief overview of some medications. It is not meant to review all the risks and benefits associated with the medications but rather to serve as a starting point for open and regular discussions with your physician. We do not cover all the possible uses, warnings, side effects, or interactions with other medicines or supplements. This information should not be used as medical advice for individual problems. Always talk to your doctor before taking any medication or supplement.

## 1. BETA BLOCKERS

Activation of the nervous system results in an increase in heart rate and in blood pressure. Beta blockers block this activation, decreasing the rate and force at which the heart pumps blood into the blood vessels. These medications can be used to lower blood pressure and to treat angina and chronic heart disease, heart failure, irregular heart rhythms, and heart attack. Beta blockers can sometimes cause fatigue, dizziness, difficulty sleeping, a slow heart rate, a rash, cold hands and feet due to reduced blood flow to the limbs, and shortness of breath in patients with asthma. Examples of some commonly prescribed beta blockers include Coreg (carvedilol), Inderal (propranolol), Lopressor (metoprolol), Tenormin (atenolol), and Toprol-XL (metoprolol).

## 2. DIURETICS

Diuretics decrease the amount of water in the bloodstream by increasing urine output. As a result, they can lower blood pressure by reducing fluid throughout the body and dilating blood vessels. These medications are used to treat high blood pressure as well as heart failure. Diuretics can cause you to feel lightheaded or dizzy (especially when you change position, as in going from sitting to standing), weakness, and fatigue. Your doctor may want to monitor certain blood tests because some of these medications can affect your potassium level and other blood chemicals. Examples of some of the commonly prescribes diuretics include Diulo (metolazone), Diuril (chlorothiazide), Hydro-chlor (hydrochlorothiazide), HydroDIURIL (hydrochlorothiazide), Hygroton (chlorthalidone), Zaroxolyn (metolazone), Aldactone (spironolactone), and Dyrenium (triamterene).

## 3. ACE INHIBITORS

Angiotensin converting enzyme (ACE) inhibitors block the conversion of a hormone in the body into a substance that increases salt and water retention. ACE inhibitors allow blood vessels to dilate and the heart to pump blood to the body more effectively. These medications are prescribed for treatment of high blood pressure and heart failure, as well as for patients after a heart attack and those with diabetes. Your doctor will monitor blood tests while you are on this medication because sometimes the potassium levels may increase and your kidney function may be affected adversely. Some patients may develop a persistent and nagging cough. If this happens to you, talk to your doctor. Other side effects include lightheadedness, dizziness, and rash. Rarely a patient will get swelling of the lips, tongue, and throat, which can interfere with breathing. If you develop these symptoms call 911. Examples of some commonly prescribed ACE inhibitors include Accupril (quinapril), Aceon (perindopril), Altace (ramipril), Capoten (captopril), Lotensin (benazepril), Monopril (fosinopril), Prinivil (lisinopril), Vasotec (enalapril), and Zestril (lisinopril)

## 4. ANGIOTENSIN II RECEPTOR BLOCKERS

Angiotensin II receptor blockers (called ARBs) act by blocking a substance that causes blood vessels to narrow. As a result, blood vessels relax, which reduces blood pressure. These medications also decrease the amount of salt your body retains, which further helps lower blood pressure. These medications are used to treat high blood pressure and heart failure, as well as in patients who cannot take ACE inhibitors and diuretics.

ARBs can cause dizziness and lightheadedness, but they do not cause a cough. Blood tests will be taken by your doctor, as potassium levels may increase and your kidney function will need to be monitored. Examples of some commonly prescribed ARBs include Atacand (candesartan cilexetil), Avapro (irbesartan), Benicar (olmesartan medoxomil), Cozaar (losartan), Diovan (valsartan), and Hyzaar (losartan).

## 5. CALCIUM CHANNEL BLOCKERS

Calcium channel blockers are drugs that slow the amount of calcium that enters the cells in blood vessel walls and heart muscle. Calcium channel blockers cause muscle cells to relax and blood vessels to dilate, reducing blood pressure and the force and rate of the heartbeat. These medications can be prescribed for treatment of high blood pressure, irregular heart rhythms, or coronary artery disease. Calcium channel blockers have different side effects depending on which medication your doctor prescribes; some can cause dizziness, nausea, or swelling of the legs, while others can cause a slow heart rate. Talk to your doctor about possible side effects. Examples of some commonly prescribed calcium channel blockers include Cardizem (diltiazem), Isoptin (verapamil), Norvasc (amlodipine), Plendil (felodipine), Procardia (nifedipine), and Sular (nisoldipine).

## 6. STATINS

HMG-CoA reductase inhibitors (or statins) block an enzyme that is involved in the formation of cholesterol and, as a result, significantly lower the LDL (bad cholesterol); they also can mildly improve HDL (good) cholesterol and triglyceride levels. These medications decrease your risk of heart attack and death from heart disease. Some patients can develop muscle aches and liver problems while on these medications. Your doctor will monitor your blood tests, and you should report any new symptoms. Examples of some commonly prescribed statins include Crestor, Lescol, Lipitor, Mevacor, Pravachol, and Zocor.

# 7, FIBRATES

Fibrates (some examples are fenofibrate and gemfibrozil) are cholesterol medications that lower triglyceride levels and increase
HDL (good cholesterol levels). Fibrates can decrease your risk of a
heart attack. These medications have side effects that can include
upset stomach, gallstones, and sometimes liver problems. Your
doctor will monitor your blood tests; report any new symptoms to
your doctor. Examples of some commonly prescribed fibrates are
Lopid and Tricor.

# 8. OTHER LIPID-ALTERING MEDICATIONS

Zetia (ezetimibe) is a cholesterol-lowering medication that
decreases cholesterol absorption in the intestines. Side effects may
include abdominal pain, back pain, diarrhea, and joint pain. Nevertheless, any symptoms you develop on medications should be discussed with your doctor. Another type of LDL cholesterol–lowering
medication are the bile acid sequestrants, such as cholestyramine,
colestipol, and colesevelam. These medications bind bile acids in
the intestines. To make more bile acids, the liver must convert more
cholesterol, which lowers the level of cholesterol in the blood. These
medications can be used alone but are most effective when used in
combination with other cholesterol-lowering medications. Bile acid
sequestrants are not absorbed into the body and therefore do not
have many of the side effects seen with the other cholesterol medications absorbed by the body. The most common side effects are
abdominal pain, bloating, constipation, and excessive gas. Vytorin is
a popular lipid-lowering medication that combines a drug for
decreasing absorption of cholesterol (Zetia) with a drug that
decreases the body's manufacture of cholesterol (Zocor).

Niacin is one of the B-complex vitamins, and in large doses, niacin lowers LDL (bad cholesterol) and raises HDL (good cholesterol) levels. Niaspan is a prescription medication with the appropriate amount of niacin for cholesterol treatment. The most common side effect is flushing, which can be limited by ingesting an aspirin one hour before taking the medication and by taking the medication with a small amount of yogurt or applesauce. Other more common side effects may include diarrhea, dizziness, itching, and rash. As with all medication, side effects can occur, and any new symptom should be discussed with your doctor.

## 9. ASPIRIN

Aspirin acts to prevent heart and stroke problems by reducing the risk of small blood clots in both men and women. Studies have shown a low dose of aspirin (61–162 mg) each day decreases the risk of recurrent heart events in women with known heart disease. Aspirin also appears to help prevent heart disease and stroke in women who have at least one risk factor and/or are sixty-five or older. As with all medications, there can be side effects and/or interactions with other medications. You should talk to your doctor before starting any over-the-counter medication or supplement, including aspirin. As an example, if you are taking ibuprofen, aspirin may be less effective and may increase your risk of intestinal bleeding.

## 10. OTHER BLOOD THINNING MEDICATIONS

These medications act by preventing blood clots from forming in the blood vessels. Coumadin (warfarin) is one of the most important drugs in this category. (We discuss Coumadin in multiple pertinent sections of this book). Examples of some other commonly prescribed blood thinners also include Plavix and Heparin. There are many medications, herbal products, supplements, vitamins, and dietary changes that can interfere with these drugs. It is important to let your doctor know all medications, over-the-counter supplements, and vitamins you are taking, as well as changes in your diet.

# Chapter
# 8
# HERBAL AND NATURAL SUPPLEMENTS: HOW EFFECTIVE AND SAFE ARE THEY?

Herbal or natural supplements can all have side effects, interactions, or potent reasons why they should not be taken. Every woman—especially if she is considering becoming pregnant or is pregnant—should talk to her physician about any over-the-counter substance she is taking. The information below is a brief overview of some common supplements. It is not meant to review all the risks and benefits associated with the individual supplements but rather to serve as a starting point for open and regular discussions with your physician. We do not cover all the possible uses, warnings, side effects, or interactions with other medicines or supplements. This information should not be used as medical advice for individual problems. Always talk to your doctor before taking any medication or supplement.

## 1. OVERVIEW

**M**any women (and men) think taking natural herbs, vitamins, and over-the-counter supplements will be more healthful for their heart than the prescription medications ordered by their physician. However, unlike medications given by prescription from the doctor, herbs and vitamin supplements do not go through a stringent evaluation process by the Food and Drug Administration (FDA). As a result, the quality and amount of a supplement may vary from preparation to preparation as well as between manufacturers. It is very important to tell your doctors about any herbal or over-the-counter supplements you use. This will help to ensure coordinated and safe care. Below are some commonly used natural and over-the-counter supplements.

## 2. BLACK COHOSH

This herb has been used to treat hot flashes, night sweats, vaginal dryness, and symptoms of menopause. Studies are mixed on whether black cohosh relieves menopausal symptoms, and investigations to address this question are ongoing. It is vital to inform your healthcare providers about any herb or dietary supplement you are using, including black cohosh.

## 3. COENZYME Q10 (COQ10)

This is a fat-soluble, vitaminlike substance. CoQ10 depletion is thought to be involved in the muscle pain some patients develop when taking cholesterol-lowering medications called statins. However, there are no well-designed studies to support this claim at this time.

## 4. EPHEDRINE AND EPHEDRA (MA HUANG)

The main active ingredient in ephedra is ephedrine—a substance that stimulates the nervous system and heart. Ephedra has been shown to cause high blood pressure, palpitations, irregular heart rhythms, fast heart rates, heart attack, and sudden death. Using ephedra may worsen heart disease, kidney disease, sleep disorders, and diabetes. According to the FDA, there is little evidence of ephedra's effectiveness except for perhaps some short-term weight reduction, but the increased risk of heart problems and stroke outweighs any benefits. Use caution when considering this supplement, and always discuss it first with your doctor.

## 5. FISH OIL

Dietary oily fish (salmon) and fish oil supplements have been shown to decrease sudden cardiac death; the American Heart Association recommends eating oily fish at least twice a week.[1] Fish oil supplements at high doses lower triglyceride levels but may raise levels of LDL cholesterol. Doctors usually recommend high-dose fish oil treatment only for people with very high triglyceride levels. As with all supplements, talk to your doctor first. The supplement may interfere with medication and/or worsen some medical conditions such as diabetes.

## 6. FLAXSEED

Studies of flaxseed to lower cholesterol levels show mixed results.[2] Some studies suggest that flaxseed may benefit people with heart disease. But not enough reliable data are available at this time, and studies are ongoing to better answer this question.

## 7. GARLIC

The most commonly cited uses of garlic are for high cholesterol, heart disease, and high blood pressure. Three well-designed research studies of garlic for lowering cholesterol levels found no effect.[3] Some research suggests that taking garlic may slow the development of heart disease or stroke, but more studies need to be done. It is still not certain whether taking garlic can lower blood pressure slightly, since the research results are mixed. Garlic, however, can act like aspirin and slow the ability of blood to clot. Let your doctor know if you are taking garlic, especially if surgery is planned.

## 8. GINKGO BILOBA

This herb may be useful in patients with peripheral vascular disease (disease of the vessels in the legs) by increasing the distance they can walk. However, because of concerns about the research designs and lack of FDA regulations for herbal supplements, the American College of Cardiology and the American Heart Association guidelines concluded that benefit is not well enough established for *ginkgo biloba* to be recommended for peripheral vascular disease.[4] Ginkgo can also increase bleeding risk, so people who use it or expect to have surgery should talk to their doctor.

# 9. PLANT STANOLS AND STEROLS

Plant stanols and sterols may act by blocking the absorption of cholesterol in the intestine. They are found as components of fruits, vegetables, vegetable oils, nuts, seeds, legumes, and grains. They are also available in commercially prepared products. Daily consumption of approximately two thousand milligrams per day can lower LDL (bad) cholesterol by 6–20 percent; intake above twenty-five hundred milligrams per day adds minimal benefit.

**Plant stanol and sterol content of food and supplements**

| Source | Plant Stanol and Sterol Content |
|---|---|
| Benecol Margarine Light | 850 mg/tbsp |
| Smart Balance Omega Plus Buttery Spread | 450 mg/tbsp |
| Smart Balance Omega Plus Light Mayonnaise | 100 mg/tbsp |
| Take Control Margarine Light | 1700 mg/tbsp |
| Nature Valley Healthy Heart Granola Bar | 400 mg/bar |
| Minute Maid Heartwise Orange Juice | 1000 mg/8 oz |
| Nature Made Cholest-Off | 450 mg/capsule |

# 10. RED YEAST RICE

Red yeast rice has been shown to lower LDL (bad) cholesterol and triglycerides while increasing HDL (good) cholesterol. It has been evaluated in clinical trials as a cholesterol-lowering agent and found to cause significant reductions in total cholesterol, LDL cholesterol, and triglycerides and an increase in HDL cholesterol.[5] The clinical evidence strongly suggests that red yeast rice is an effective natural product for controlling serum cholesterol. It should be avoided in pregnant women and in women planning on getting pregnant, people with liver problems, individuals younger than twenty, and those already on a cholesterol therapy with a statin. Always talk to your doctor before starting any herbal or vitamin supplement.

## 11. SOY PROTEIN

Soy protein contains isoflavones, which mimic the action of estrogen. The Nutrition Committee of the American Heart Association reports that isoflavone supplements do not appear to be of benefit and should not be taken with a goal of improving cholesterol. Soy foods (tofu, soy butter, and soy burgers) are likely to have beneficial effects on cholesterol and heart health because they are low in saturated fats and high in unsaturated fats—and soy products often can be used to substitute for meats, dairy products, and other high-cholesterol foods.

## 12. ST. JOHN'S WORT

Some studies suggest that St. John's Wort is beneficial for treating mild depression. However, it is not a proven therapy, and if symptoms persist, women should follow up with their doctors.[6] This herb can interfere with several drugs. Therefore, talk to your doctor before starting this or any supplement.

♥ ♥ ♥

As the bottom line, we caution that, while considered more "natural" than manufactured drugs, herbs and supplements are largely unproven for the putative benefits postulated, and each poses dangers of its own. If you are about to have cardiac (or other) surgery, please, please be sure to tell your surgeon and your anesthesiologist about each and every one of your supplements—in order to avoid excess bleeding, adverse interactions with anesthetic agents, and other potentially life-threatening consequences of your seemingly innocuous supplements.

# STRESS, DEPRESSION, AND ANGER: IS YOUR HEART AT EMOTIONAL RISK?

## 1. THE EFFECTS OF STRESS ON A WOMAN'S HEART AND HEALTH

Research has shown that sudden emotional stress, particularly in women, can trigger a severe but reversible heart muscle weakness similar to a heart attack, as noted earlier. The condition has been called broken heart syndrome, and the cause appears to be stress hormones. People respond to stress in their lives by releasing adrenalin and other stress hormones into the bloodstream. Sudden and significant stress in some women causes the release of large amounts of these chemicals, which results in the heart muscle's becoming stunned. Women typically feel chest pain and shortness of breath during the event. Luckily, the heart muscle usually does recover with medical treatment within a few weeks without specific interventions such as angioplasty, stents, or surgery. It is very important to call 911 with any symptoms of a heart attack, including a "broken heart" scenario.

Stress has long been linked to ill health, but importantly there is a direct link between stress and metabolic syndrome. Metabolic syndrome is a group of factors that put a woman at high risk for heart disease. Metabolic syndrome includes the presence of three of the following:

- a waist measurement greater than thirty-five inches (in women)
- a high blood pressure (systolic blood pressure greater than 120 mm/Hg and/or diastolic blood pressure greater than 80 mm/Hg)
- a low HDL (good cholesterol) level (less than 50 mg/dl in women)
- a high triglyceride level (greater than 150 mg/dL)
- a high fasting blood glucose level (greater than 100mg/dL).

Women with chronic stress are more likely to suffer from metabolic syndrome.

The INTERHEART study was an investigation of risk factors for heart disease, including stress, that compared patients with a first heart attack with those who did not have a heart attack.[1] For the former, stressful events frequently preceded the attack. The stresses included marital separation or divorce, loss of job, retirement, business failure, violence, major family conflict, personal injury, illness, death or major illness of a close family member, death of a spouse, or other major stress. Stress is part of our daily lives, but the degree and our bodies' response are important, as shown on the facing page.

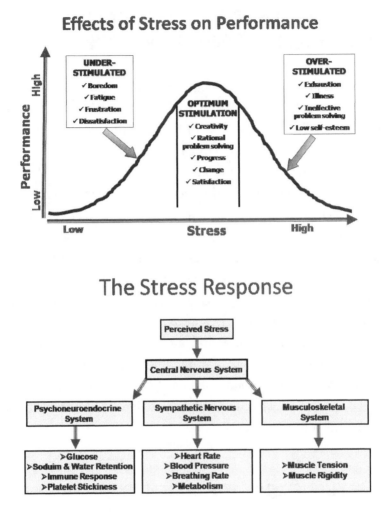

Heart attack is not the only major, life-threatening acute cardiac event directly correlated with acutely stressful life circumstances. Our group has demonstrated exactly the same causal relationship between specific stressful events in one's life and a catastrophic cardiac event known as acute aortic dissection. In this syndrome, the aorta, the main artery of the body, is split into layers by an advancing wave of blood under high pressure.

## 2. DEPRESSION—OFTEN OVERLOOKED BUT A SERIOUS RISK TO WOMEN

But it is not just stress; other emotional factors such as depression, hostility, and anger have been associated with the development of heart disease. The lifetime risk for major depression is 7 to 12 percent for men but as high as 20 to 25 percent for women. Depression is an illness that involves not only mood and thoughts but also the physical body, affecting appetite, sleep, self-esteem, and life in general. Without treatment, symptoms can last for weeks, months, or years. Appropriate treatment, however, can help most people with depression. Depression and depressive symptoms are also very common in patients, especially in women, recovering from a heart attack and coronary artery bypass surgery. Studies have shown serious depression develops in approximately 20 percent of patients after a heart attack.[2] Depression after a heart attack increases a patient's risk of dying. Cardiac rehabilitation programs, medications when indicated, and increased social support may help improve symptoms of post–heart attack depression and should be recommended to all patients.

## 3. METHODS AND TREATMENTS TO HANDLE STRESS

There are many ways to manage stress, and the following stress management strategies will require practice to be effective.

### Deep Breathing

Often, when we are stressed, we take small, shallow breaths and often hold our breath without even realizing it. When you feel stress building—perhaps while driving in traffic or during the workday—take two minutes for yourself. Try the following: take twelve *deep*, slow breaths. Breathe in through your nose and out through your mouth. Learn to relax with deep, controlled breathing. This technique, practiced once or twice a day for ten to twenty minutes, will result in a relaxation response that decreases stress, as shown below.

## The Relaxation Response

- ♥ Is a deep state of rest
- ♥ Is different from sleep
- ♥ Decreases heart rate, blood pressure, and breathing rate
- ♥ Helps neutralize the effects of the stress hormones
- ♥ Allows your body to return to normal
- ♥ Allows you to regain your ability to cope with stress

## Protected Time: You Are Important and So Is Your Health, So Take Time for YOU.

In general, women are nurturing and, as a result, often try to meet everyone else's needs. It is time to make sure you are not short-changing yourself. Set aside protected time to take care of the inner you, even if it is only fifteen to thirty minutes. Do something you enjoy that relaxes you, such as sitting in the yard reading a book, listening to music, taking a hot bath, going for a walk, or just taking a cat nap.

## Guided Imagery:
## A Vacation without Leaving Your Desk!

Sit quietly and think of a pleasant memory or place you have visited. Close your eyes and imagine this place where you feel happy and relaxed. Guided imagery is a technique used, through thoughts and suggestions, to lead your imagination toward a relaxed, focused state. You can learn this technique from educational tapes or an instructor. Studies have shown guided imagery can decrease stress, decrease heart rate, and lower blood pressure.

## Exercise

Exercise can be a very effective means of reducing stress. Try to find an exercise activity you enjoy and make regular time for it. Going to the gym, walking, swimming, gardening, or playing with your children can relax you: the body and mind work together. Exercise has been shown to increase the release of chemicals called endorphins that result in your having more energy and feeling relaxed. Here are some creative ways to overcome obstacles to getting started with your exercise program:

- Weigh the costs and benefits; when the benefits outweigh the costs, you are ready to make your commitment.
- Start slowly and set small, achievable goals.
- Choose an activity that you enjoy and that is convenient.
- Schedule a specific time and day for exercise.
- Preplan your day, such as having workout attire in your car.
- Evaluate and chart your progress.
- Strive for consistency; you cannot reinforce irregular behavior.

- Learn from your setbacks but do not focus on them.
- Get a support system.
- Surround yourself with positive reinforcement, such as people who want to help you with your goals.
- Be a positive role model for others.
- Have a backup plan for unexpected challenges.
- Preplan travel, such as calling to make sure the hotel has a fitness area or a safe, convenient place to walk.
- Keep an open mind and try new things.
- Continue to educate yourself about the benefits of exercise.

If you have never exercised, or if you have risk factors for, or have been diagnosed with heart disease, it is important to talk to your doctor before starting an exercise program.

## Sleep

All of us need adequate sleep to reenergize both the mind and body. Any amount of sleep deprivation will diminish our mental performance. And studies have shown that stress can disrupt sleep patterns. To minimize sleep problems, try to keep a regular bedtime and wake-time hour—this means on weekends too! Try to make your bed and bedroom a cool, quiet, and restful environment.

Avoid alcohol because it will not remove the cause of your stress but only masks the problems. Prescription medications for sleep should be taken only on the advice of your doctor. Many can be addictive.

## Now Some Final Words from Dr. Caulin-Glaser's Heart to Yours to Get You Through the Day:

- Forgive and forget. Yes, I said forget! Life is too short to focus on the negatives; we all have made mistakes, especially if we have lived our lives with passion.
- Delight in who and where you are—respect the time given to you and use it well.
- Laugh often—it is a natural stress reducer.
- This inspirational quote from an unknown author appears above my desk: "Work like you don't need the money; love like you've never been hurt; and dance like you do when nobody's watching."

To summarize, the links between stress and heart disease continue to be demonstrated through scientific research. How does stress have this effect? First, stress often leads to unhealthy behaviors, including smoking, alcohol use, overeating, and exercising less. Second, stress has its own effects on the heart, such as increased blood pressure, heart rate, and stress hormone levels. It makes sense to avoid stress where possible and to learn to manage stress where it cannot be avoided—by learning more about and using the techniques we briefly reviewed in this chapter.

# Chapter
# 10
# CARDIAC TESTING

## 1. WHAT IS THE BEST TEST FOR WOMEN AND WHY?

**W**henever you have symptoms that may be heart related, you need to undergo cardiac testing to confirm their origin.

Your cardiac evaluation begins with what we call the history and physical exam.

Your doctor will talk to you about any history you may have of heart attack, stroke, high blood pressure, high cholesterol, and the like. He will ask you about classic cardiac symptoms, such as **angina** (chest pain) and **shortness of breath**. He will also ask you if you get **lightheaded** easily or if you have ever **passed out** (the medical term for passing out is syncope). He will inquire whether you feel **palpitations** (flutterings) of your heart. These are all classic indicators of heart problems. Angina signals coronary artery disease. Shortness of breath may indicate congestive heart failure, inadequate blood flow to the heart, or valvular heart disease. Lightheadedness or syncope may indicate disturbances of the rhythm and rate of your heart, specifically too slow or too fast a heart rate. So without even listening to your heart—just by speaking to you— your doctor gets a good sense of how well your heart meets the needs of your body. If you have none of these symptoms, it is unlikely that you have advanced heart disease.

The doctor will ask you about any history of heart disease in your family members, as this can indicate your own susceptibility to heart disease.

Next your doctor will examine your heart.

- *Pulse exam.* The doctor starts by feeling your pulse. He can tell the rate of your heart, its rhythm, and about how much blood is being pumped with each beat. He will also feel pulses in other regions besides your wrist. If a good pulse is felt, that means blood is reaching those parts of your body and that there are no severe intervening arterial obstructions. Classically, your doctor will feel the pulses in your wrists, in your neck (carotid), in your groin (femoral), and at your feet (dorsalis pedal and posterior tibial). The character of the upstroke of the arterial pulse in the carotid region provides a good indication of whether there is any blockage of the aortic valve (aortic stenosis); such blockage would produce a delayed, blunted upstroke to the pulse.
- *Blood pressure.* The doctor or nurse will check your blood pressure. We like to see a blood pressure below 140/90, or in some cases even lower. Too high a blood pressure damages your arteries, leading to heart attack, stroke, or even kidney failure or congestive heart failure.
- *Feeling your heart.* This is called palpation. The doctor will place his hand over what we call the apex, or tip, of the heart. This is located in the crease under your breast, toward the left edge of your breast. If the maximal impulse is found too far left, that can indicate that the heart has enlarged excessively. The doctor's hand may be able to detect a vibratory sensation called a "thrill"; this usually indicates severe valve disease. It is the equivalent of a murmur, but it is so severe that it can actually be felt.

- *Listening to your heart.* This is the aspect of the exam most familiar to patients. The doctor learns a great deal about your heart by listening. He can tell if the heart is beating rhythmically, as it should. He will listen for a heart murmur, which can be a sign of valve blockage or leakage. You can aid the exam by removing all layers of clothing from your chest so that the doctor can get his stethoscope directly onto the skin overlying your heart. The heart tones are distant and subtle, and the doctor needs every advantage in listening to them. Resist the temptation to talk while the doctor is listening to your heart. If you talk, he cannot hear your heart, which is drowned out by the intense reverberations of your speech.
- *Listening to your lungs.* Believe it or not, the lungs reflect the status of your heart. The doctor listens for rales, or fine crepitations, which signal congestive heart failure, due to backup of water into your lungs. He also listens for decreased sounds of breathing, which can signal fluid deposited around your lungs in the chest cavity, which is called pleural effusion.
- *Checking your ankles.* Your doctor will check your ankles for buildup of fluid (called edema), a sign of congestive heart failure.

By means of the history and physical exam, your doctor will get a very clear picture of your cardiac status. Your doctor may elect to perform additional tests, which are discussed below.

# 2. ELECTROPHYSIOLOGIC TESTING

## Chest X-Ray

The regular chest x-ray tells the doctor a tremendous amount about your heart. The x-ray clearly shows the overall outline of your heart.

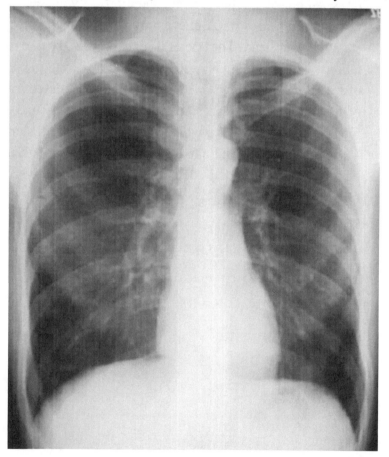

She can tell if your heart is enlarged—and sometimes she can even make out which chamber is most affected by the enlargement. The x-ray also clearly shows the amount of fluid that may be backed up in your lungs. A smaller amount indicates congestive heart failure, and a large amount signifies an advanced heart failure state called pulmonary edema.

## Electrocardiogram (EKG)

Nearly everyone is familiar with the electrocardiogram. This test, which reads electrical signals from sticky electrode pads attached to the skin under your left breast and on both arms and both legs, reveals a great deal about your heart.

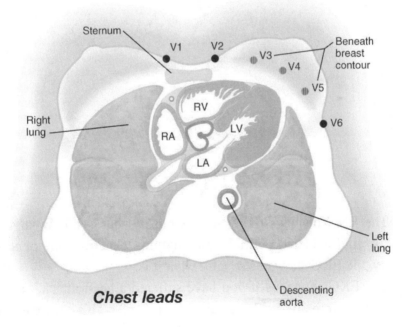

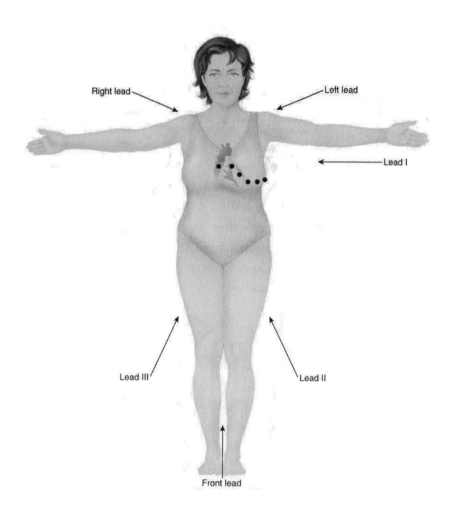

The EKG displays the exact rhythm of your heart. What we usually find is called normal sinus rhythm. If there is any abnormality, the EKG shows us exactly what it is.

The EKG shows us if you have suffered a heart attack, either recently or in the past. (See figure 2.9 on p. 62). This shows up as abnormal downward deflections, or Q-waves. The EKG does not directly display the pumping strength of your heart or the action of the valves of its heart.

## Echocardiogram

The echocardiogram has become a very commonly included part of a cardiac evaluation—almost part of the extended physical exam. As the machines become smaller and smaller some researchers have speculated that a miniaturized echocardiographic probe may be the stethoscope of the future. The echocardiogram, or "echo" for short, uses reflected sound waves—like sonar—to make pictures of your heart. This is completely safe. You or your daughter likely had many echo exams of the uterus and fetus during pregnancy. The echo depicts the walls and chambers of your heart with great precision. We can measure each chamber precisely, calculate the fluid pressures inside your heart, and evaluate the pumping strength of your heart very accurately—all with this entirely noninvasive testing modality. Many patients consider the echo fascinating, as it is totally painless, and you can watch your heart in action as the exam is done. The echo calculates an ejection fraction for your heart—this is an index of how powerfully your left ventricle, the main pumping chamber of your heart, is contracting. Even though this is expressed as a percentage, normal is not 100 percent; rather, normal individuals have an ejection fraction of 50 to 55 percent. The echo can even be used as a stress test to evaluate whether you have occult coronary artery disease, as we will see below. Women have a somewhat higher resting ejection fraction than men. (This is but one of many reasons that Dr. Elefteriades says, "Women are stronger, smarter, and much better looking.") With exercise, however, women increase their ejection fraction somewhat less than men do.

## Screening CT Scan

You may see advertisements in magazines and newspapers encouraging you to go for an "ultrafast CT scan" to see if you have silent coronary artery disease. Such CT scans are often part of for-profit, freestanding imaging centers. The principle behind such scans is that, with severe arteriosclerosis, calcium ultimately becomes deposited in affected coronary arteries. This calcium can be detected very well by CT scanning. The appropriate role of these scans is controversial, as severe blockages may not always be calcified and, conversely, calcified lesions may not always harbor severe blockages. You might consider such a test if, based on your cholesterol or a positive family history, you are very concerned that you may harbor silent coronary artery disease. You do not even need an outside doctor's prescription to go for one of these for-profit scans. But if you have such a test, be sure to let your doctor know the results. Remember that severe blockages may not always be calcified and thus can elude the screening CT scan.

CT scanning is improving rapidly in its technical accuracy, especially with the new generation of 64-slice scanners, which can visualize coronary arteries noninvasively to an accuracy never before realized or anticipated. Even as this is written, 128-slice scanners are on the horizon. It is quite possible that within five or ten years, CT scanning may replace angiography (invasive dye injection) in many cases.

## IMT Testing

In the same vein, so to speak, another advertised service at for-profit centers is the so-called intimal-medial thickness (IMT) test. You may find IMT studies being offered for a small fee at your local shopping mall. This test looks at your carotid arteries—the large arteries in the neck—to see if their walls have thickened. This is a quick, painless, noninvasive, echo-based test. If your carotid arteries are not thickened, this indicates that arteriosclerosis is not present to any significant degree in your body, likely not in your coronary arteries either. A normal thickness score is a good sign. An abnormal score, which suggests deposits in the wall of the carotid arteries, leading to increased thickness, is a general indicator of arteriosclerosis in your body. A positive score requires alertness to manifestations of disease affecting your brain or heart; more invasive and specific further imaging may be recommended. We have no objection to your having an IMT test by a reputable company, provided that you review the results with your own doctor.

# 3. STRESS TESTING

Stress testing, as the name implies, puts a load on your heart and looks for signs of inadequate blood flow under conditions of high load. Stress tests, designed to detect coronary artery disease *before* it causes a heart attack, are of paramount importance in women for a number of reasons. Anginal symptoms are more variable in women and more difficult for the physician to recognize. About 40 percent of heart attacks in women are fatal, at least at the time of the famous Framingham study.[1] Moreover, 67 percent of cardiac deaths in women have occurred in individuals who did not previously know that they had heart disease.

The multiple kinds of stress tests are detailed below.

## Ordinary Stress Test

The original form of stress testing, still practiced and valuable today, involves your walking on a treadmill while doctors and technicians monitor your pulse, blood pressure, and EKG. They exercise you quite strenuously, close to the highest heart rate attainable at your age, so that they can impose an extreme load on your heart. They look for abnormal rhythms of your heart under stress, a drop in blood pressure (which normally goes up with exercise), and especially for changes in the EKG pattern of your heart. These are all indicators of what we call *ischemia*, or inadequate blood flow to the heart under stress. They especially look for what is called *ST segment elevation*, as seen in figure 2.9 (heart attack) on page 62. (The ST segment is a normally straight, flat portion of the heartbeat, as displayed on the EKG.) This ordinary stress test is about two-thirds sensitive in picking up coronary artery problems. (About one-third escape detection.) If the test is abnormal, it is about three-quarters accurate in its indication of coronary artery disease (with the other quarter representing a false test, or a false positive, as it is called). In general, stress testing is not as accurate in women as in men.[2] Estrogen effect, lower blood count, and other factors have been implicated in this difference.[3]

## Stress Echocardiogram

This test uses the echocardiogram in addition to the regular EKG to monitor your heart's function as you exercise. This adds accuracy to the results, as the doctors and technicians actually see your heart in action, while they follow its electrical signals. They look for decreased contractile strength in vulnerable regions of your heart that may be provoked by exercise. They divide your left ventricular wall into segments (usually sixteen), and they grade the motion of each. Normally, the segments move more strongly with exercise than at rest. A segment or segments that fall behind indicate the presence of coronary artery disease. The stress echo exam is substantially more accurate than an ordinary stress test without echo. If you are not able to exercise, your heart may be stimulated by a powerful drug called dobutamine, which exaggerates the differences between the normal and abnormal segments.

## Nuclear Stress Test

This stress test looks at your heart with a nuclear "camera" while you exercise. It provides highly accurate images of your heart's pumping strength under stress, actually visualizing the blood flow to your heart.

Despite the ominous sound of the name—nuclear stress test—the actual exposure to radiation from the injected dye is small. This test is often combined with drugs (dipyridamole, adenosine, or dobutamine) to increase the stress. This test is highly sensitive and specific—that is, it doesn't miss many true cases of coronary artery disease, nor does it create many false positive results. If your test is negative, you are no more likely to have a cardiac event than the normal population of individuals; there is less than a 1 percent-per-year likelihood that you will suffer a heart attack in the year to come. If you have a positive test, the likelihood of such an adverse event is nearly 25 percent, unless you have corrective treatment.

The one problem with a nuclear stress test in women, as noted earlier, is that the image of the heart can be obscured by the left breast, especially in large-breasted women. This situation is depicted in figure 10.6. In fact, if your breast shifts in position during the various images, this can mimic the defect of a real area of insufficient blood flow. Although nuclear stress testing is especially prone to this problem, the ordinary stress test and the echocardiographic stress test are not. If you have large breasts, you might ask your doctor about the possible confounding of images if he plans to refer you for a nuclear stress test.

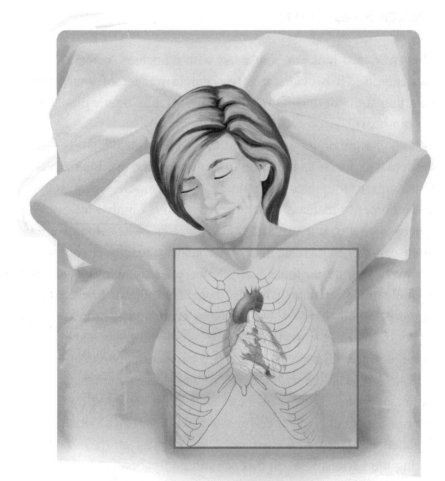

## PET Scanning

PET scans, widely available only recently, constitute another modality for detecting abnormalities of blood flow to your heart. This method is quite promising and may see more clinical use in the near future. PET scanning has an uncanny ability to visualize and measure actual coronary artery blood flow via a noninvasive test.

# 4. ANGIOGRAPHY

Angiography is the "gold standard" test for coronary artery disease.

This test is considered invasive because it requires a needle be placed into a main artery (usually the femoral artery in the leg) and a catheter be threaded into the heart to inject dye directly into the openings of the coronary arteries. This test is also called cardiac catheterization. Despite being invasive, cardiac catheterization is very safe. Mortality or major complications (such as stroke or heart attack) are exceedingly rare. This test is extremely accurate: it depicts the anatomy of the coronary arteries in great clarity and detail, permitting any significant blockages to be brought to light.

**Table 10.1. Potential Tests For Coronary Artery Disease In Women**

| Test | Invasive? | Sensitivity | Specificity | Special Issues In Women |
|------|-----------|-------------|-------------|--------------------------|
| Stress test (EKG based) | Noninvasive | 56% | 75% | Less accurate in women |
| Stress ECHO (5) | Noninvasive | 88% | 84% | |
| Nuclear stress test | Mildly invasive (radioactive dye injected) | 90% | 90% | Breast shadow may obscure images in women |
| Angiography | Invasive (catheter, dye) | 100% | 100% | |
| PET imaging | Noninvasive | | | Emerging, but promising modality |

Note: *Sensitivity* refers to the ability of a test not to miss affected individuals. *Specificity* refers to the likelihood that an individual who appears, on the basis of the test, to be affected, really is affected.

With the historical questioning, the physical examination, and the noninvasive and invasive tests described above, your doctors can obtain quite a precise picture of the presence or absence, and the severity, of your heart disease.

# Chapter
# 11
# PROCEDURES AND SURGERY: WHY WOMEN DO MORE POORLY THAN MEN

For women whose heart disease is not controlled by medications, one of several well-proven interventions may be required, either in the catheterization suite (catheter-based interventions) or in the operating room (surgical procedures). These are discussed on the following pages.

Let us look at the available techniques for controlling heart disease when drugs are not adequate.

## 1. ANGIOPLASTY

Most women have heard of angioplasty, which is also termed percutaneous coronary intervention (PCI). The not-so-affectionate terminology is "plaque busting." The word percutaneous means "through the skin"—that is, without an incision. The frequency of this procedure has grown from one thousand per year when first introduced to over four hundred thousand per year currently in the United States.

This entire procedure is done via a needle stick, usually in the large artery in your groin (specifically, in the crease between your lower abdomen and your thigh). In this form of therapy, a cardiac catheterization and coronary angiogram are performed first. This may be done on an emergency basis, if you have presented with unstable angina or a heart attack in evolution, or as a part of a scheduled procedure. Within your heart, the artery with the plaque and thrombus causing the angina or heart attack are identified. Then, a balloon dilation, or angioplasty, is performed—most often augmented by delivery of a metal stent. (A stent is a wire mesh that looks like the spring in a ballpoint pen. The wire structure is intended to keep plaque from growing toward the center of the vessel and once again narrowing the flow channel.)

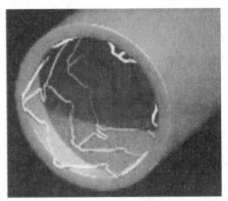

The balloon is inflated by fluid under pressure in the catheter. The results are immediate and dramatic: the offending artery is widened, assuring adequate blood flow to the affected cardiac muscle.

If you have a television or an Internet connection, or if you read any newspaper or magazine, you must have heard the recent controversy about so-called drug-eluting stents. A stent by itself is effective in the short term, but the stented site often narrows in the long term. Medical science was looking for a method to prevent that long-term narrowing, known technically as late restenosis. The answer seemed to have been found in the drug-eluting stents. These stents are coated with a drug that prevents scar tissue from forming as the body's reaction to the foreign metal of the stent. Actually, the drug comes from the family of medications used to prevent the body from rejecting transplanted organs. The drug coating gradually "leaches" out from the stent, providing a durable prevention of local scarring.

Drug-eluting stents have markedly reduced the incidence of in-stent restenosis—repeat narrowing within the stented area—to about the single-digit percentage range. This has been a major advance in angioplasty techniques.

Recent information, however, indicates a chink in the armor, so to speak—almost as if the benefit of drug-eluting stents was too good to be true. In the last several years, some patients with drug-eluting stents have died suddenly from heart attacks. We have found that these are related to sudden thrombosis (clotting) of the stented artery. It appears that this occurs mainly in patients who stop taking the anti-platelet drugs prescribed after drug-eluting stent placement. Specifically, a powerful drug called Plavix, which makes your platelets nonsticky, preventing clotting, is an essential adjunct after placement of a drug-eluting stent. This drug may be maintained long term. When it is stopped abruptly, then clotting and a heart attack can occur.

It appears that the rate of sudden closure of the drug-eluting stent site accounts for about a 2 percent-per-year death rate. This is a very large number. Many, if not most, of these sudden closures and deaths are related to cessation of the powerful blood thinner Plavix. Many cardiologists specializing in stent treatment have moved back to ordinary (non-drug-eluting) stents, especially under the close scrutiny of the Food and Drug Administration (FDA). In fact, you should discuss with your heart doctor whether coronary artery bypass may be a preferable alternative to placement of a drug-eluting stent in your case. This is a topic of debate between cardiologists (who perform stenting) and cardiac surgeons (who perform the bypass procedure). Each specialist, cardiologist or surgeon, generally believes most fervently in his modality of treatment. The stent market also makes this a multibillion-dollar industry for manufacturers, so there is a strong push for stent therapies. It appears that the recently confirmed trouble with stents argues in favor of the traditional coronary artery bypass operation, which provides reliable, durable results. We have definitely seen a drop-off in stent therapy and a recrudescence of coronary bypass. Please discuss the two options—stent therapy and coronary artery bypass surgery—in detail with your general doctor, your cardiologist, and, preferably, a cardiac surgeon.

### Risk of Angioplasty in Women

Simply stated, women have more complications after angioplasty than men do. Women develop a split ("dissection") in the artery undergoing angioplasty more commonly than men.[1] Women have a heart attack more frequently after angioplasty than men. Women die more frequently after angioplasty than men.[2] These higher complication rates may be related to the smaller size of women's coronary arteries, to the arteries' greater tendency to spasm after manipulation, and to the simple fact that women are older when their coronary artery disease is diagnosed. Still, even in women, the chance of a heart attack or death after angioplasty is low: about 3 percent.[3]

## 2. CORONARY ARTERY BYPASS SURGERY

We are very much in favor of the coronary artery bypass operation (affectionately called CABG—pronounced "cabbage"). CABG, simply put, is one of the best-proven, most effective interventions in the history of medicine. And keep in mind, we are partial to CABG because Dr. Elefteriades has performed over three thousand of these procedures in his career.

## Who Needs a CABG Operation?

There are several indications for the coronary artery bypass operation. Indication is the medical term for the appropriate scenario in which a certain type of therapy should be applied.

The first set of indications has to do with functional criteria, that is, issues of how you are getting along, or coping, with your coronary artery disease. If you have no angina or a stable, tolerable pattern of angina, you may not need a bypass operation. If, however, your angina is disabling, so that your quality of life is adversely affected or you cannot carry out daily activities—like work, recreation, or family life—a bypass operation may be appropriate for you. A bypass operation is also appropriate for patients who have an unstable anginal pattern, one that is increasing in frequency or severity.

If you are in the hospital with a heart attack in progress or a threatened heart attack, a bypass operation may be essential to keep these events controlled—by supplying more blood flow to the threatened areas of heart muscle.

The second set of indications has to do with anatomic criteria, that is, issues of extent and severity of the actual blockages. If you have severe disease of the most important artery of the heart—the left main coronary artery—you need surgery. Likewise, if you have disease of all three arteries of the heart and you have had significant damage to your heart from a prior heart attack, you need bypass surgery. If you have less disease, say, of only one or two arteries, and you feel well and get along, you may not need a bypass operation.

Our coronary arteries, like everything else in our bodies, are overdesigned. The amount of blood flow through your vessel is not impaired until a blockage equals or exceeds 60 to 75 percent. Thus, when we talk about significant blockages in one, two, or three arteries, we mean only blockages exceeding those percentages.

Your doctor may bring other factors to bear on the decision for bypass surgery. For example, if you did very poorly on your exercise test, with a fall in blood pressure, abnormal heartbeats, severe EKG changes, or abnormalities on imaging (suggesting a large amount of heart muscle at risk), a bypass operation may be vital. Similarly, if these worrisome changes were brought on early in the stages of exercise, that suggests bypass surgery may be essential.

**Indications for coronary bypass surgery**

| Functional indications | Anatomic indications |
| --- | --- |
| 1. Threatened heart attack | 1. Left main lesion |
| 2. Incapacitating angina | 2. Three-vessel disease, with prior |
| 3. Unstable anginal pattern | heart attack |

| Worrisome findings on stress testing |
| --- |
| 1. Trouble early in test |
| 2. Fall in blood pressure |
| 3. Major EKG changes |
| 4. Large area at risk on images |

The decision for or against bypass may at times be simple and at other times more complex. You need to discuss this issue carefully with your cardiologist and your heart surgeon.

## How the Bypass Operation Is Done

There are two widely used conduits for construction of bypass grafts. The original is the vein from your leg, which we call the greater saphenous vein. This runs along the inside of your thigh and calf, from groin to ankle. If you find the bump that represents the inner side of your ankle, what we call the medial malleolus, you may be able to see the vein just in front of that bump. If you stand up, the vein will fill with blood, which appears as a bluish streak. You may be able to feel the vein full of blood when you stand or sit with your feet on the floor. This is the superficial vein of your leg, carrying only a small amount of the total blood flow returning from your leg to your body. (Remember, veins carry blood back to the heart from other organs. Arteries carry blood from the heart to other organs. The bypass operation does *not* use any arteries from your leg.) The deep vein from your leg carries 95 percent of the blood flow. After we use the superficial vein for your bypass operation, the deep vein will take on the small extra burden.

Nowadays, at most centers, the saphenous vein is harvested with a scope through two small incisions, rather than the three-foot linear incision we used to make. You will hardly even know that your leg has been touched during the operation. The small scar on the inside of your thigh, near the knee, is nearly imperceptible.

The other common conduit, very popular since 1983, is the internal mammary artery, which runs on the inner aspect of your breastbone, just to either side. Both men and women have two of them. These arteries supply blood to the ribcage, the breastbone, and the breasts, for which the artery is named. This is a great conduit, with exceptional long-term results, as discussed below.

Women may worry that harvesting the mammary artery may have an adverse effect on the breast, but this is simply not the case. Although the mammary artery is named for the breast that it supplies with blood, no detriment to the breast occurs following the surgery. The breast has an abundant network of blood vessels besides the mammary artery, which continue to supply all the blood flow required— even after the mammary artery has been borrowed for use on the heart.

Figures 11.1a and 11.1b illustrate the bypass operation schematically, and figure 11.2 shows actual photographs from the operating room, some taken with extreme magnification.

♥ ♥ ♥

Usually, the connections of the conduits to the coronary arteries, which we call the distal anastomoses, are constructed first. Distal means farther along an anatomic structure, and anastomosis means hookup. The tiny artery is incised with a blade, then the incision is extended with scissors. The length of the opening is about five millimeters (one-fifth of an inch), and the width is about one to two millimeters (one-tenth of an inch). The conduit and the artery are attached by about a dozen and a half stitches taken with a single running suture. The suture is pulled up to parachute the conduit down onto the artery. Note that the conduit is sewn to an opening made in the side of the coronary artery. The artery is not cut in half. The diseased artery is not removed. This would be both impossible, and unnecessary. The hookup is done beyond the last blockage, thus "bypassing" the blockage and providing free blood flow to your heart muscle.

After the hookup to the coronary artery is done, the vein is connected to the aorta, or the main artery of the body, so that the vein may receive blood flow to carry to your heart. This is called the proximal, or upper, anastomosis, because it is located upstream to the heart. This hookup is done by punching a five-millimeter (one-fifth of an inch) hole in the aorta and again suturing with a running stitch taken many times through both structures. The end of the vein is sewn to a hole in the side of the aorta.

If the bypass is done with the mammary artery, no proximal anastomosis is necessary, as nature has already done that. The mammary artery comes already attached to a great source of inflow, the subclavian artery—the main artery to your arm.

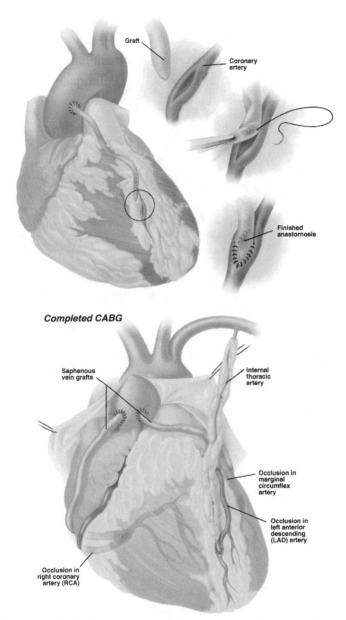

Figures 11.1a and 11.1b. The coronary bypass operation, illustrated. Part a shows how we open the coronary artery and do the hookup with a vein. Part b shows the completed operation. Note this represents a "triple" bypass, with two vein grafts and one mammary graft, all of which are shown.

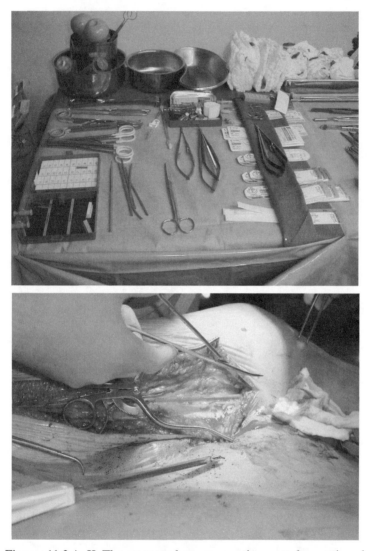

Figures 11.3 A–K. The coronary bypass operation, actual operative photographs. Part A shows the table of fine instruments used for the delicate suturing of the coronary vessels. Part B shows the vein being harvested from the thigh. In this figure, the head of the patient is to your left and the foot is to your right. You can see the knee just above the surgeon's scissors. Part C shows the vein harvested and being prepared on the back table. Part D shows the heart exposed for surgery. Part E shows the tubings from the heart-lung machine being placed into the heart chambers. Part F shows the important LAD artery being incised for hook-up. Part

G shows a close-up of this incision. The LAD is running left-to-right across the photograph. Part H shows an extreme close-up of the suturing process. Note that several stitches have been taken between the open coronary artery below and the mammary artery above. The needle is being passed outside-in through the wall of the mammary artery. Re-member that the mammary artery you are seeing is only 1.5 mm in diameter (like the lead in a pencil). The suture material itself is just visible to the naked eye. Part I shows the mammary artery being "parachuted" down into place onto the coronary artery, after a number of sutures have been placed. Part J shows the mammary now in place. You can see that additional sutures need to be placed to complete the hookup. Part K shows the completed anastomosis. The mammary artery is now connected to the LAD coronary artery. The LAD can be seen as the thin white structure that runs toward the lower right hand corner of the photograph. All operational photographs courtesy of author.

Part C

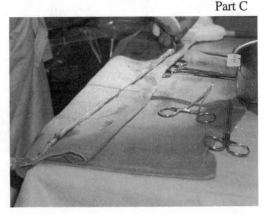

Part D

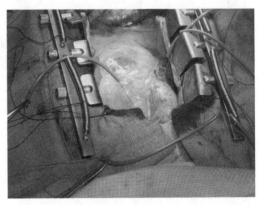

Part E

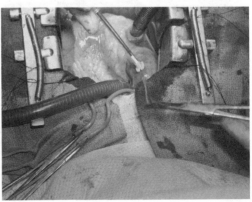

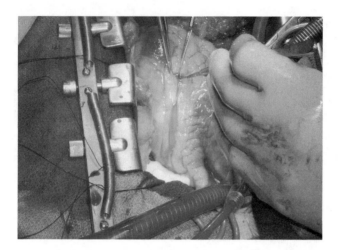

Part F

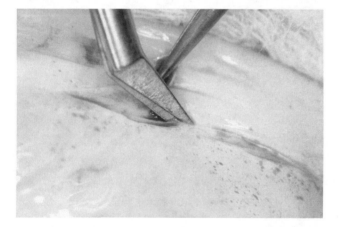

Part G

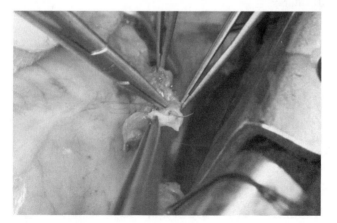

Part H

Part I

Part J

Part K

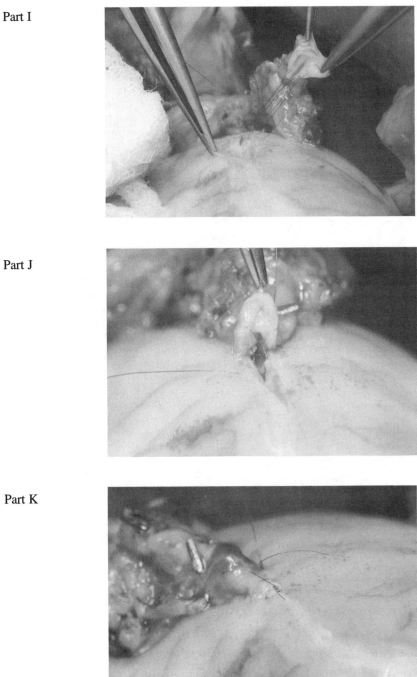

The CABG operation is usually performed with your heart stopped and your body on what we call the heart-lung machine. (In the very first utilization by surgical pioneer C. Walter Lillehei, a baby's mother was used as the "heart-lung machine" to propel the baby's blood while the baby's own heart was stilled; this was accomplished by a set of tubes linking the circulations of the baby and the mother.

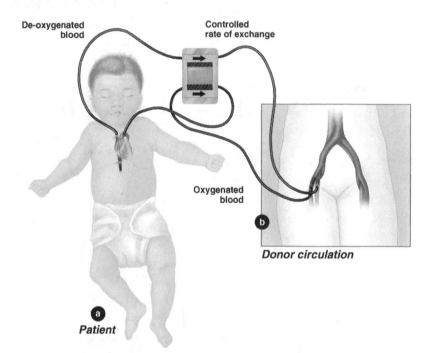

De-oxygenated blood

Controlled rate of exchange

Oxygenated blood

Donor circulation

Patient

Over the decades, the mechanical heart-lung machine has been incredibly refined, and the device itself and the state of being on this machine, "on bypass," if you will, has become very safe, so you need not fear it. It will easily support you for hours at a time, if needed. In some cases, usually simpler bypass operations in patients with good, large target arteries, the CABG operation may be performed without the heart-lung machine, with the heart still beating. This technique is effective as well.

The CABG operation does have risks. Some patients may not survive; some may suffer a stroke; and others may have bleeding or infection or other problems. In the United States, the in-hospital risk of death or serious complication after CABG averages at only 2 percent for low-risk patients. See more about risks specifically for women in the paragraphs below.

## How Long Will My Bypass Operation Last?

First of all, not all individual bypass grafts constructed at operation will function effectively. One month after the operation about 95 percent of the bypasses will "take"—that is, carry blood and remain open. This percentage is about the same for all conduits, that is, for both vein grafts and for the mammary artery. Note that the patient may be fine if one or more individual bypasses have closed.

It is not surprising that the early function rate is not 100 percent. Few things are 100 percent in life. When you think of all the factors that must play themselves out just right for an individual bypass graft to function, it actually becomes surprising that so many vein grafts do function well. The target artery must have a soft area where the bypass may be placed. The target area must irrigate a sufficient distribution of heart muscle for there to be a relatively large, high velocity flow of blood through the bypass. The vein or other conduit must be of good quality and tolerate the mechanical trauma of being harvested and stored (albeit briefly) until use. All eighteen or twenty sutures must be perfectly placed, so none encroaches on the opening, or lumen, through which blood flows. This is no mean feat, as all these sutures are placed into an artery that is one to two millimeters in diameter, or about the thickness of the lead in a no. 2 pencil. Imagine placing so many fine sutures around the perimeter of such a small structure. In addition, no clots must form at the slightly irritated zones where the stitches cross the wall of the artery or vein. Similar favorable events must play themselves out at the end where the vein is attached to the aorta at its upper, or proximal, end. Furthermore, the length and lie of the graft, after both ends are attached, must be perfect and smooth, without kinking or tension or excess length. (It is really an art, rather than a science, for your surgeon to accomplish all this.) The body must avoid forming excess swelling at the sites of connection of blood vessels. Later on, the body must avoid depositing excess scar tissue at the sites of hookup of blood vessels. As you may know, a scar in the skin thickens. If the same happens internally where the vein is attached to the coronary artery, a narrowing, and possible closure, of the bypass graft will occur. Thus, the excellent 95 percent patency (actively functioning) rate of bypass grafts is a miracle of sorts, which to this day fascinates us, despite our own application of this operation in thousands upon thousands of patients.

Now, let's move on to the ten-year point. Are the bypasses still open? Well, for the vein grafts, about 40 percent will have closed and 60 percent will still be open. Why will some have closed? The reason is recurrent arteriosclerosis. More disease may attack your vein graft or the artery to which it attaches, leading to closure. Not all bypasses are so affected. In fact, even within the same single patient, some vein grafts may become diseased, while others remain pristine. We do not understand the reasons for such differences.

At the ten-year point, however, the situation is much different for your mammary graft. Nearly the same 95 percent that were open at one month are still open at ten years. The mammary artery is essentially immune to arteriosclerosis. We do not know why this is true, but we are glad that it is so. The favorable behavior of the mammary artery used as a bypass graft is so impressive that some surgeons have speculated that nature put it on the inside of the chest wall so that it could be used for this very purpose.

The good news does not end there. Let's go out to fifteen and twenty years after your bypass. Believe it or not, the same 95 percent of mammary grafts that were patent (open) and functioning at one month, and at ten years, are still open and pumping at fifteen and twenty years. Those mammary grafts just keep on pumping. They are almost eternal, even if disease in your original coronary arteries progresses.

The accompanying chart shows the percentage of grafts of the two kinds still functioning at various times after the bypass operation. The superiority of the mammary bypass operation is clearly evident.

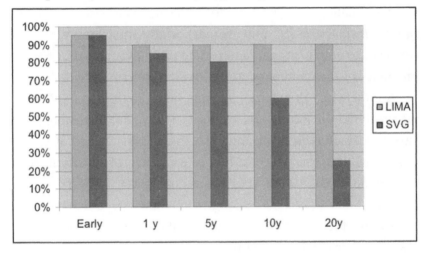

LIMA = left internal mammary graft. SVG = saphenous vein graft. Constructed from data appearing in J. F. Sabik III, B. W. Lytle, E. H. Blackstone, P. L. Houhtaing, and D. M. Cosgrove, "Comparison of Saphenous Vein and Internal Thoracic Artery Graft Patency by Coronary Stystem," *Annals of Thoracic Surgery* 79, no. 2 (February 2005): 544–51.

If the mammary artery is so wonderful, why do many patients have only the left mammary artery used, when there is also a right mammary artery? That is a good question. The right mammary does not perform as well as the left as a conduit for the bypass operation. Why in the world would this be? Didn't nature make the two mammary arteries equal? Indeed, it did, but, the left mammary is an easy reach to the most important artery on your heart, the left anterior descending (LAD). Part of the reason that the left mammary bypass does so well is that it is placed to the LAD, which keeps a large volume of blood flowing through the graft at all times.

The right mammary does not reach as well to important targets, since your heart is located a bit more to the left side of your chest. Because it is a more difficult reach, the right is not used as frequently as the left mammary artery in the coronary artery bypass operation. Because the right mammary graft is used to secondary arteries, smaller and with less flow, its results are not as strikingly superb. In many cases, however, especially for younger patients, we may use both mammary arteries, to take advantage of the innate immunity of the mammary artery to arteriosclerosis.

Are there any drawbacks to using both the right and left mammary arteries in the bypass operation? Yes. The breastbone will have less blood flow for healing if both arteries are used. If you are a diabetic, you can expect a higher incidence of infection of the breastbone incision after your bypass operation, from a 2 percent likelihood to a 4 percent. As long as you understand this, your surgeon may still choose this option for the benefits of two arterial grafts in your long-term future.

If your vein grafts do close over the long term, is it possible, you may wonder, for the CABG operation to be performed a second time? Yes, the bypass can be done a second time, if necessary. It is more difficult and dangerous the second time for many reasons. You will be older. Your cardiac structures will be stuck together inside—what we call adhesions—because of the irritation to internal membranes by the first operation. The location of the bypass on your coronary arteries will be "second choice," so to speak. There are also many other technically complicating features. But experienced centers can offer second-time operations with confidence and good expectations.

The operation is sometimes performed a third time, if necessary, and, rarely, a fourth. In one case, we performed a sixth-time coronary artery bypass operation. The benefit becomes more limited with these multiple performances, and the dangers mount swiftly with the number of reoperations.

How is the number of bypasses I need determined? Each of us is born with three major arteries that run on the surface of the heart and provide the heart muscle with blood. These are one to three millimeters in diameter, or about the size of the lead in a pencil to the size of the refill in your ballpoint pen. A patient can have single-, double- or triple-vessel disease. It is important to recognize that each of these main arteries divides into literally innumerable smaller tributaries, like the branches of a tree. One can count any number of arteries. We customarily count only the three major branches and their major tributaries.

You will hear your cardiologist or surgeon use the names of the blocked arteries or the ones bypassed. You can review the anatomy of the coronary arteries again in figure 2.1 on page 38.

The origin of the coronary artery to the left side of the heart is called the left main coronary artery. This, in turn, divides into the left anterior descending coronary artery (or LAD) and the circumflex coronary artery. The former is the single most important artery of your heart, supplying 40 percent of your heart's total blood flow, as noted. This one is called the "widow maker," in recognition of the devastating impact of a sudden occlusion (closure) of this vital tributary. This left anterior descending coronary artery courses down the very front of your heart. The circumflex runs around the left side to supply blood to the side, or lateral, wall of your heart. The right coronary artery rises separately and runs along the right side to supply the bottom, or inferior, wall of the heart.

You will also come across the names of the branches of the coronary arteries. The branches of the left anterior descending coronary artery are called diagonals when they run to the side of the main vessel, or septals when they course directly deep into the heart muscle. The branches of the circumflex coronary artery are called the marginals. The main branch of the right coronary artery is the posterior descending coronary artery, or PDA. You can use the diagram in chapter 4 to locate the arteries that your doctors talk to you about. This diagram will also serve to indicate what regions of your heart are irrigated by which arteries.

The pain related to blockages in the different arteries is felt in the center of your chest. The right coronary artery doesn't cause pain on the right, nor the left coronary artery on the left. The body cannot discriminate between insufficient blood flow caused by the different arteries.

Your surgeon will bypass all the arteries that have major blockage and are big enough and soft enough to take a graft. More is not necessarily better. Bypassing an artery that is too small or too diseased may actually increase your risk of adverse events. This is where your surgeon's training and experience come to bear—in creating the "work of art" that is your bypass operation.

## Effectiveness of the Bypass Operation

About three-fourths of patients will have complete relief of their angina. Many of the remainder will glean substantial relief in terms of frequency or severity of angina. Some few patients do not benefit for a variety of reasons. Their bypasses may not all function well, or even a small artery, not big enough to bypass, may cause severe angina. In general, however, the bypass operation is very effective in relieving angina symptoms.

It is worthwhile to note that up to 15 percent of patients may require some angioplasty "touch up work" in the first year after bypass surgery.

If you are feeling well, without chest pain or significant shortness of breath with exertion, it is likely that your bypasses are working fine. How you feel is the single overridingly most important factor in the assessment of your bypass operation. Your cardiologist may also do a stress test periodically to assess your heart's response to exercise.

Your bypass operation is just plumbing, albeit very delicate plumbing. The coronary artery bypass has absolutely no effect on the chemistry of your body that caused the deposits to develop in the first place. Your cholesterol and other lipids will resume their prior levels when your diet stabilizes after surgery. Controlling your cholesterol and other risk factors will be just as crucial after your operation as before. Without controlling your risk factors, you may not glean as much benefit from your new bypasses. Controlling these risk factors ensures that your bypasses will function as long as possible.

Far and away the most important risk factor for you to control is cigarette smoking. If you smoke, your bypasses will close. It is that plain and simple. You must never smoke another cigarette after your bypass operation. You will, by necessity, have been smokefree for all the days that you were in the hospital. Take this opportunity to continue your smokefree state, and your bypasses—as well as your overall health—will benefit greatly. The benefits to your family will be great, too. You will ensure that you will be around to enjoy their company for the longest time possible.

While you are in the hospital it may be helpful for your family to carry out some supportive maneuvers regarding smoking cessation. Your family can clean the home environment, dry clean the drapes, steam clean the rugs, and the like, to remove the smell of smoking from the house. The car interior can be detailed for the same reasons. We want you, the patient, never, ever to have another cigarette after your return home.

Not only is the coronary artery bypass procedure a proven form of treatment, but some authorities, including us, feel it ranks as *one of the most proven modalities of treatment in the history of humankind.* The procedure has been performed since the mid-1960s. For decades, more than four hundred thousand such operations have been performed yearly in the United States alone. The procedure has been tested every which way but sideways. The bypass procedure has been studied in many carefully designed multicenter randomized clinical trials—the most stringent mechanisms for evaluation of any treatment modalities. Time after time, these evaluations have shown that the procedure works, and works very well. It has been shown that: (1) Bypass surgery is safe. (2) The individual bypass grafts actually work. (3) Patients' symptoms (usually angina) are relieved by the bypass operation. (4) Patients' lives are prolonged by the operation. (5) The bypass operation can restore some of the pumping strength of the heart that has been lost over years of heart disease. (6) Benefits of the coronary artery bypass operation are very durable.

Another testimony to the effectiveness of the coronary bypass operation is that results of most, if not all, of the formal trials have been interpreted in whole or in large part not by surgeons but by cardiologists. This should eliminate most potential undue favorable bias, as coronary bypass is not a procedure that cardiologists perform; thus they have no inherent reason to wish to see its benefits exaggerated. In fact, cardiologists have multiple conflicting technologies that they themselves offer, so their strong support of the coronary artery bypass operation speaks volumes in and of itself.

## Results of CABG in Women Specifically

You might not expect a gender difference in CABG results, but there is no question that, over the years, mortality from CABG has consistently been higher in women. Every experienced cardiac surgeon knows that a woman may have very small, very delicate coronary arteries—which may challenge the technical limits of this amazing operation. A target coronary artery needs to be large enough to be grafted and strong enough to hold sutures. On rare occasion, these conditions may not be obtainable; this situation is seen more frequently in women than in men. Smaller body size is definitely a factor. In fact, when careful studies have teased apart the impact of a patient's sex and the impact of body size (regardless of sex), it has become apparent that the real risk factor is actually body size, not the patient's sex. Because women are smaller, they show a greater mortality risk from CABG. Please recognize, however, that this difference in risk between men and women is small (2.7 percent vs. 1.8 percent risk of death), and CABG remains a very safe operation for both men and women.[4]

## 3. VALVE SURGERY

A common joke among medical practitioners is that cardiac surgeons do only three operations: coronary artery bypass grafting, mitral valve replacement, and aortic valve replacement. While this is an exaggeration, valve surgery is a very important part of what we do. Valve disease, from congenital malformations, wear and tear of age, or infection, is quite common, especially in women. In fact, over two-thirds of patients discharged from the hospital after care for valve disease are women.[5] Many valve diseases, including rheumatic heart disease and mitral valve prolapse, predominantly affect women—they are about one and a half times more common in women. In this section, we address your valve surgery in particular.

## When is Valve Repair Necessary?

If you have major narrowing (stenosis) or leakage (regurgitation) of your aortic or mitral valves, you may well need surgery. This is certainly the case if you feel poorly—shortness of breath, lightheadedness, or an inability to perform the tasks of everyday life. In some cases, your doctor may recommend valve surgery for your narrowed or leaky valve, even if you feel reasonably well.

As the science of valve assessment and replacement becomes more advanced, we realize that in many cases, the left ventricle, the main pumping chamber of the heart, may be deteriorating even while the patient continues to feel well. This is especially true with the "leaky" conditions—mitral regurgitation and aortic regurgitation. If this deterioration progresses too far, the risk of eventual surgery may become excessive, and the benefit may be limited, as the deterioration may be permanent, even after a good new valve is placed. The reason is that the regurgitant lesions place a large volume load on the left ventricle. (See chapter 1 for the reference to the Sisyphus-like burdens of leaky valves.) The left ventricle stretches and stretches to keep an adequate amount of blood flowing forward despite the leaky valve. The stretched muscle is overloaded and suffers damage, both temporary and permanent.

Your doctor may recommend surgery, even if you feel well, if serial studies (usually ECHOs, see above) show that your heart is progressively enlarging. Likewise, if your studies show that the pumping strength of your left ventricle is falling, even to the lower ranges of normal, this is evidence of the severe impact from your leaky valve. If your valve is not replaced promptly, your well-being and long-term survival will be compromised. Your doctor may also do a stress test. If your left ventricle pumps more weakly under stress, that indicates that your heart is being unduly damaged by the leaky valve. In such a circumstance, prompt surgery is vital.

In certain instances, your heart valve may be leaking so badly that surgery is recommended immediately, without further studies. We grade the severity of leakage on a scale of I to IV. If you have grade IV leakage of your aortic or mitral valve, surgery will likely be recommended, as only bad things will happen without surgical intervention.

Please keep in mind that most patients with valvular heart disease learn to adjust to it. You may think you feel well, but you may have subtly limited your lifestyle and activities to adjust to your more limited heart capacity. You may take the elevator more than before and do less walking up the stairs. You may walk slowly rather than hustle. You may ride rather than walk around the golf course. Many patients tell us how very much better they feel with a new valve, even though they thought they felt "well" before.

Remember that your leaky heart valve is a *mechanical* problem. No medication, no length of delay can make your valve function better. No medication can prevent the eventual damage to your heart. A severely leaking heart valve is a mechanical problem that requires a mechanical solution: surgery.

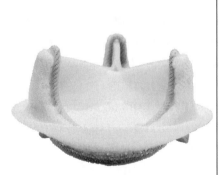

Figure 11.4. An animal valve (Carpentier-Edwards PERIMOUNT aortic heart valve). Image courtesy of Edwards Lifesciences, Irvine, California. Reprinted with permission.

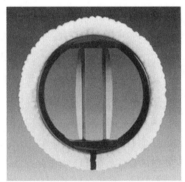

Figure 11.5. A mechanical valve (St. Jude valve). Regent™ Mechanical Heart Valve: Regent™ is a tradmark of St. Jude Medical. Reprinted with permission from St. Jude Medical™, © 2008 all rights resered.

## Kinds of Replacement Valves

There are two general types of artificial heart valves, animal (or tissue) and mechanical. Each type has specific advantages and potential liabilities.

Animal valves generally are made from tissues from pigs (called porcine valves) or cows (called bovine valves). (See figure 11.4).

The pig valves are generally removed directly from animals grown specifically for this purpose, then mounted on delicate hardware that supports the valve and incorporates a sewing ring to facilitate its securing to the patient's heart. These valves are natural in that they functioned as valves in the animal from which they were removed.

In the case of valves from cows, the tissue is actually removed from the cow's pericardium, the strong material that makes up the sac that surrounds every mammal's heart. This raw material, like a thick plastic wrap in consistency, is precisely and delicately fashioned into humanmade leaflets, three of which are incorporated to make up a valve. The finished product has a cloth sewing ring. All this construction is done by the manufacturers, and the valves come prepared and ready for implantation off the shelf.

For both pig and cow valves, the animal colonies are carefully monitored to be certain that the strains are healthy.

Occasionally, we may use a valve taken from an expired human being. These are called homograft valves. The valves are carefully inspected to make certain that they function well, and the donors are screened for communicable diseases. Further, the valves are fully disinfected and frozen. Their function and longevity are comparable to those of animal valves.

The mechanical valves are completely humanmade. They are produced from a material called pyrolite carbon, which is the same substance from which artificial diamonds are made. This material is very hard and smoothe, so that it does not attract blood clots. Several manufacturers make valves from this material, under different product names. (The best known is the so-called St. Jude valve. See figure 11.5.) These valves also incorporate a cloth sewing ring.

All the valve types come in a variety of sizes. An operating room contains a complete range of sizes in stock. The process is analogous to shoe sizing. Every individual has a different size annulus (valve ring) into which the new valve needs to be placed. A sizing instrument is placed into the annulus in your heart to measure the size you need. That sized valve is taken from the shelf for your use. Women's valves are usually considerably smaller than men's.

The two types of valves—animal and mechanical—have their own intrinsic benefits and liabilities. Animal valves have the wonderful advantage that they are "blood friendly" by virtue of their being biological material; for this reason, they do not promote clotting and thus do not require blood thinners. This is a very important plus. However, the great disadvantage is that they wear out in due course, since they are not being kept alive and are not replenished or restored by your body. The collagen in the valves is what gives them their structure. It can bend, to open and close, only so many times. We explain this to our students by analogy of an expired credit card. Many users tear up the card to avoid its unauthorized use. Those of you who have tried this, however, know that it has to be flexed and unflexed many, many times before it breaks. It is the same with the collagen in your animal valve; this can take millions upon millions of heartbeats, but, eventually, it will give way.

By the way, animal valves cannot be rejected by your body. Unlike a heart, a kidney, or a liver, the animal valves are not alive, and for this reason cannot be rejected. Only the biological scaffolding of the original valve persists in your body—not any living animal cells that are prone to rejection by your own body's immune mechanisms.

Animal valves can be expected to last well over a decade. In some cases, they can last fifteen or even twenty years. There is some evidence that the newest pericardial valves (cow tissue) last longer than any prior animal valves ever developed. One interesting fact is that animal valves last a long time in older patients and much shorter times in the young, but we do not know why. In an adolescent or a young adult, for example, an animal valve may break down even within the first five years.

Mechanical valves, by virtue of not being biologic in origin and composition, are not as friendly to the blood and tend to attract and promote microscopic blood clots. For this reason, lifelong administration of blood thinners is generally recommended for patients with mechanical heart valves. (See also chapters 1, 8, and 15, regarding Coumadin.) The great advantage of mechanical valves is their durability. One type (the so-called St. Jude valve) has been in use for thirty years and has not yet worn out. Over one million patients have received this valve. Structural failures of any kind have been almost unheard of. What will happen after thirty years medical science simply cannot say, but three decades is a very, very long time in medical care, especially where the heart is involved.

Regarding the need for blood thinners, it is essential to point out that its common for patients who receive animal valves to require blood thinners for other reasons. Some surgeons use blood thinners for a brief period even after placing biological valves. In patients with valvular heart disease, atrial fibrillation, an irregular rhythm of the upper chambers of the heart (see above), is quite common and blood thinners are frequently used for patients with that rhythm. This rhythm requires blood thinners so that clots do not form in the irregularly contracting upper chambers of the heart. This situation can negate the advantage of animal valves vis-à-vis blood thinners.

Younger women are always concerned about the effect of Coumadin on their menstrual flow. In general, menstrual flow does increase substantially because of the use of Coumadin, but this is rarely a substantial health concern. The advantages of having a mechanical valve that can last a lifetime usually trump the inconvenience of heavier periods until menopause. As discussed in other sections of this book, use of Coumadin during pregnancy is problematic, and, if you plan on more childbirth, this factor has to be taken into account.

## Implanting the Valve in Your Heart

The first step in implanting a new valve in your heart is to gain access to that valve. These operations are usually done through what we call a median sternotomy incision, which runs up and down the center of your chest and right through your breastbone (see figure 11.6). This leaves only a thin scar in the middle of your chest. In men, this is covered well by their chest hair. In women, the top of this incision may show slightly when you wear an open collar or a low neckline.

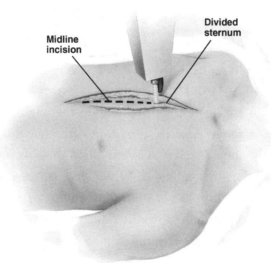

Figure 11.6. The median sternotomy incision.

This incision may sound bad, but actually the median sternotomy is easy, quick, and quite comfortable for you post-operatively. Next, we need to put you on the heart-lung machine in order to stop your heart and open the appropriate chamber. The heart-lung machine takes the place of your heart and lungs while we work. To access your aortic valve, we make an incision in the aorta. To access your mitral valve, we make an incision in the left atrium (see figures 11.7a and 11.7b).

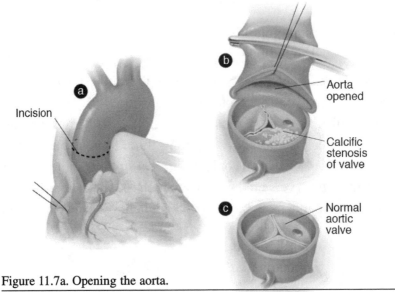

Figure 11.7a. Opening the aorta.

The first step in replacing your valve is to remove the old, diseased valve. This is excised sharply by scissors or blade. This leaves a soft but strong fibrous ring, called the annulus, to which the new valve is sewn. A series of sutures are placed through the annulus, usually about twelve to twenty, and then passed through the cloth ring of the artificial valve. When these sutures are tied, the valve "parachutes" into place within the annulus of your heart. A water-tight, secure attachment results. This process is shown in the figures below. The process is quite similar in both the mitral and aortic positions (see figure 11.8).

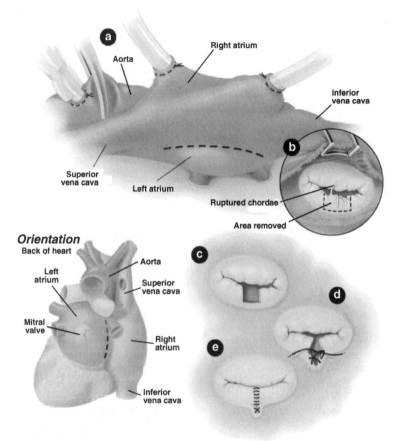

Figure 11.7b. Opening the left atrium and repairing the mitral valve.

In time, your body will reinforce this attachment by growing tissue into the interstices in the cloth sewing ring of the valve. However, the secure attachment of your valve will always depend on the sutures. The material of these sutures, reassuringly, is essentially eternal. Even decades later, the sutures appear just as strong as the day they went in.

You may have heard about delivering valves into your heart by catheter (without an incision). In the animal laboratory, some success has been achieved in incipient forays into this method. These investigational procedures have been performed to replace per-

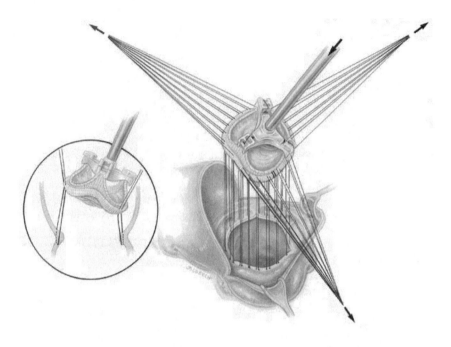

Figure 11.8. Installing a new valve.

fectly normal valves, which are not removed; the catheter-delivered valve is placed within the normal native valve. Initial clinical trials in patients too ill for conventional valve surgery are beginning. It is too early to know if this will prove a viable treatment modality, even in highly selected cases.

## Repairing, Rather Than Replacing, Cardiac Valves

In certain cases, your own valve can be repaired rather than replaced. This is most applicable to the mitral valve when it is leaky rather than narrowed. In technical parlance, repair is often feasible for mitral regurgitation.

The development of mitral valve repair represents one of the greatest advances in the history of cardiac surgery. This is largely the life's work of Dr. Alain Carpentier of Paris, France, one of the greatest surgeons in history and, arguably, the best teacher of cardiac surgery *ever*.

Dr. Carpentier's techniques permit surgeons to excise the diseased portion of the mitral valve and bring the remaining tissues back together, with very delicate manipulation and suturing, to form a properly functioning whole. Usually the leak in your own mitral valve results from the tearing of one of the fine parachutelike cords that control the movement of the delicate mitral valve leaflets.

You are *not* being shortchanged if your mitral valve is repaired rather than replaced, for there are major advantages. First, you shouldn't need Coumadin in the long term. The fine cords that support your mitral valve also support the muscle of the left ventricle, so this whole parachutelike apparatus is preserved when your mitral valve is repaired. Specifically, your heart muscle remains stronger because of this preservation, and your life expectancy is better in the long term.

On the other hand, some leaky valves just cannot and should not be repaired. In such a situation, a good valve replacement is better than an incomplete or a nondurable valve repair.

For the aortic valve, repair techniques have not been generally adopted. Also, aortic valve replacement does not carry the detrimental consequences that can sometimes follow mitral valve replacement. For these reasons, repair is, practically speaking, limited to the mitral valve.

## Living with an Artificial Heart Valve

The valve you receive, whether animal or mechanical, cannot be rejected, because it is not alive. A transplanted heart, a liver, or a kidney can all be rejected by your body because they are alive and performing active, vital functions. In contradistinction, your heart valve, while very important, is not alive and performs no active functions. It functions passively, opening or closing as your heart muscle propels blood forward. It is easy to understand that the mechanical valve, made of artificial, humanmade materials, is not living. However, even the animal valves are treated in such a way that living cells are removed and only the scaffold of collagen, a basic structural building block of the body, remains. The valve is not renewed by your body, unlike all your own tissues and organs, which are "rebuilt" regularly by your body's inherent renewal mechanisms. So you need not have any concern regarding rejection of your valve.

Your new valve can, however, become infected, and that can be very serious. Because it is an artificial part, it cannot clear bacteria from its surfaces the way your own tissues can. We teach our students that the interstices in the cloth of the sewing ring provide an environment where bacterial organisms can take hold and thrive. We use the analogy that these small crevices may serve as a "luxury hotel" for bacteria, while the surrounding blood provides "room service," with all the nutrients that the bacteria require to proliferate.

But infection is very rare on new valves. We cannot recall the last time that this occurred in our patients. These events usually reflect some type of contamination during the surgical procedure to place the new valve or some infectious event early afterward that forced bacteria into the bloodstream. You will be given antibiotics preventatively (prophylactically is the medical term) around the time of your operation to provide extra protection from such events. The likelihood of an early infection of your valve is less than 1 percent.

The only circumstance in which such infections are common occurs when the valve replacement is being performed specifically to treat a native valve that is already infected. This is called endocarditis, again from the Greek, meaning infection of the inside of your heart. In such a circumstance, you will be given antibiotics for weeks to discourage even any stray remaining bacteria from seeding your clean, new valve. Nonetheless, infection does recur with some regularity in such cases, and it's very serious and difficult to eradicate.

# 4. PACEMAKERS AND DEFIBRILLATORS

Pacemakers and defibrillators are wonderful electrical devices that can save your life—very literally. Pacemakers kick in and stimulate your heartbeat when your pulse gets too low, and defibrillators shock your heart when the rate becomes too fast.

## Pacemakers

For some patients, their heart rate may be too slow at baseline or may fall too low at specific isolated times. In general, we like to see a heart rate between sixty and a hundred beats per minute at rest.

Remember that the forward output of the heart depends on the heart rate. Generally, the faster the heart rate, the larger the forward output. By corollary, if the heart rate falls too low, the output will be insufficient.

Very few of us—predominantly only trained athletes—can maintain a good forward cardiac output at heart rates below sixty beats per minute. Thus, this represents the lower range of heart rates at which we become concerned. In fact, there is a special term for heart rates below sixty: bradycardia, meaning "low heart rate."

If your heart rate runs at or falls below sixty, it is quite possible that you may need a pacemaker. This is especially true if you have such symptoms as dizziness, passing out, or a severe lack of energy. If you have these and demonstrate sustained or episodic bradycardia, you likely need a pacemaker, which can be absolutely life-saving for you. A very low heart rate can easily and frequently be lethal. So dramatic can be the loss of consciousness related to a sudden slow heart rate that the medical term "drop attack" has been coined; that is to say, with a sudden onset of low heart rate, the patient loses consciousness and literally drops to the ground like a sack of potatoes.

You may hear your doctor talk about various types of slow heart rates. First is so-called sinus bradycardia; this means a low heart rate that originates normally in the sinus node, the heart's normal internal pacemaker. Alternatively, your doctor may tell you that you have a "first-degree heart block"; this refers to a slight delay in conduction of electrical impulses in your heart. More serious is "second-degree heart block," in which some beats are actually dropped. Most serious is "third-degree" or "complete heart block," in which all normal beats are blocked. In such a rhythm, your heart stops unless an internal accessory pacemaking tissue in your heart jumps into action—which does not always occur.

Placement of a pacemaker is usually a quick, straightforward process. That is not to say it is trivial, but it usually goes extremely smoothly and involves little or no discomfort for you. You are sedated but not fully anesthetized. Novocaine is injected just under your collarbone and a small incision made. One vein that leads to your heart is accessed, and the pacing lead is passed through that vein and positioned carefully at the tip of your right ventricle, directly inside your heart. The position is checked carefully by x-ray, and the electrical characteristics of pacing are calculated, to be sure that they are optimal. A small pocket is fashioned to accommodate the pacing unit, and the incision is closed. The pacemaker is so small—barely bigger than a silver dollar—chances are that neither you nor anyone else would even be able to tell it was there.

With the pacemaker in place, you will never, ever die of too slow a heart rate.

## Defibrillators

Defibrillators are implanted similarly to pacemakers, through an incision under your collarbone. These are a little larger than pacemakers because their battery needs to store more energy. Defibrillators are appropriate for patients at risk for very rapid heart rates, usually ventricular tachycardia or ventricular fibrillation. These are the rapid, uncoordinated rhythms you see on TV monitors, just before a patient has the electrical "paddles" applied. These rhythms usually result in cardiac arrest, but the implantable defibrillators—which are very, very effective—prevent this. If your doctor recommends one, she is worried that you are vulnerable to sudden cardiac death. She may be concerned because you have already had a bad rhythm event or because the pattern of damage to your heart makes such an event likely. Defibrillators are an extraordinary development of modern medical science and can fairly be credited with saving thousands of lives. Having an implanted defibrillator is like having a whole emergency room inside you—doctor, EKG machine, paddles—watching each and every heartbeat, ready to apply an electrical current at any time that a life-threatening rhythm occurs. Living with a defibrillator is entirely a win-win situation, as there are no common serious risks from having a defibrillator in place watching for your safety.

# 5. HEART TRANSPLANTATION

In some rare instances, the damage to the heart is so severe that no conventional treatment—medications or coronary bypass, valve replacement, or other surgical procedures—can adequately rehabilitate your heart and safeguard your life. Under such circumstances, a heart transplant may be recommended. Usually, you will have been treated for congestive heart failure for some time before a transplant is deemed necessary. Your ejection fraction (normally 55 percent, see above) will have fallen very low by this stage, usually below 20 percent. Your breathing will be labored despite water pills and other medications. You may find yourself frequently or repeatedly admitted to the hospital for difficulty breathing. Your life is in jeopardy from month to month, and a transplant is in order.

We used to say that sixty was the strict upper age limit for heart transplantation for two reasons: First, elderly patients did not do as well in the short or long term after heart transplantation. They died more frequently and had more complications than their younger counterparts. Second, there was a strong sense among doctors of an ethical imperative to allocate preciously scarce donor hearts to younger patients, who had not had an opportunity to live through a normal lifecycle.

Currently, the situation has changed somewhat so that patients over sixty can, on occasion, be considered for transplantation. Certain high-profile cases have resulted in a consensus that strict age criteria are discriminatory and not acceptable. Results of transplantation in older patients have also improved. So if your general health, other than your heart, is good and you are active and have the potential for a vigorous life of good quality, you may be considered for transplantation even if you are over sixty. Surgeons are now putting more patients between sixty and sixty-five years of age on lists for donor hearts than in the past. Beyond sixty-five, only the very rare patient should have a transplant.

For patients without associated medical problems in other organs, heart transplantation is relatively safe. About 90 percent of patients will survive the transplant operation and the early recovery phase. About 80 percent to 90 percent of patients will be alive one year after transplantation. About 50 percent to 60 percent of transplantation patients will be still be alive five years later. After that point, it is quite likely that coronary artery disease will develop in the transplanted heart, leading to death over the five- to ten-year interval following transplantation. Some patients have lived over twenty years following transplantation, but that is the exception rather than the rule. These uniquely fortunate patients probably benefited from a fortuitously favorable immunologic match with the donor.

Patients wonder whether their new heart comes from a dead person. The answer is both yes and no.

The donor heart cannot ordinarily be taken from an individual who is dead in the usual sense—that is, without a heartbeat, a pulse, or blood pressure. The heart is very sensitive to interruption of its own blood flow. If the donor were literally dead, his heart would not be of use. It would have died itself or become severely weakened.

However, the person whose family kindly donates the heart to you will be dead in another sense—specifically, *brain* dead. That is, although he will have a heartbeat, a pulse, and blood pressure, he will be unconscious, without volitional movements, and never be able to attain consciousness again. Strict criteria have been developed to ensure that the declaration of brain death is accurate, unequivocal, and permanent.

One of the biggest problems in heart transplantation today, now that effective antirejection drugs have been developed, is finding a donor organ before the waiting recipient succumbs to advanced heart failure. Most donors have suffered some type of direct brain injury, resulting most commonly from automobile or motorcycle accidents or from a gunshot wound by rupture of a brain aneurysm. In all these cases, brain death will be diagnosed only after a rigid series of observations have been unequivocally confirmed by independent observers. Because of the donor shortage, it is important for as many of us as possible to sign up in advance as potential donors in case of overwhelming injury. The wonderful operation of transplantation can take a (donor's) tragedy and turn it into the miracle of life (for the recipient).

Much research and debate, professional and in the press, has concerned the possibility of taking donor hearts from animals. Famed transplant surgeon Dr. Norman Shumway of Stanford University was asked about this two decades ago. Transplanting animal hearts is called xenotransplantation, from the Greek word *xeno*, meaning "stranger." Dr. Shumway's reply has become legendary. "Xenotransplantation," he said, "is five years away. And it always will be." Clearly, Dr. Shumway did not feel that this modality was likely to come to clinical fruition. A testament to his acumen, xenotransplantation is not much closer to clinical reality than when he made that pithy and witty remark.

The potential problems are numerous. First of all, the antigenic differences between species will pose rejection dangers far exceeding those of human-to-human transplantation. (Antigens are signature proteins on the surface of cells that identify one species and one individual as different from others; they are highly irritating when transplanted into another organism.) Engineering nonantigenic animals is currently being attempted, yet it is far from satisfactory. There is also the serious potential danger of exposing the human race to infections, especially viruses, both known and unknown, that are currently limited to other species, especially in the current AIDS era. Finally, there are ethical issues about growing animals specifically for the purpose of donating their hearts to humans.

The regulation of research and application of xenotransplantation require the input of not only scientists but also clergy, ethicists, legislators, and the general public.

## Heart Transplant Surgical Procedure

When you are undergoing a heart transplant, first, you are placed on the heart-lung machine, which substitutes for the pumping action of your heart. Then, your heart is removed. No doctor ever forgets his first sight of the empty chest cavity.

At the same time, the new heart arrives—usually brought by jet from the donor hospital. The new heart is trimmed and prepared to suit your anatomy.

The new heart is attached to your body by a series of four anastomoses, or hookups, which include the left atrium, the right atrium, the aorta, and the pulmonary artery.

The new heart is allowed at least a half hour of blood flow after attachment to your body before it is given any load. At that point, in a gradual fashion, the burden of pumping your blood is transferred from the heart-lung machine to your new heart. Your new heart always needs some support with stimulating medications until it recovers from the trauma of excision, storage, transportation, and transplantation.

## Special Issues Regarding Heart Transplantation in Women

The smaller size of women plays a role in matching a donor and recipient. This factor works in favor of female recipients, who are generally smaller than men, with less muscle mass. Thus, a female heart is smaller, on average, and less powerful than a man's heart. Therefore, special precaution must be taken in selecting a heart from a female donor for a male recipient. The converse is true, however. A male heart is usually a great match for a female patient as it is more than large and powerful enough—it's like installing an eight-cylinder engine in a car that normally has a six cylinder one.

There has been speculation that a female recipient's personality can change by virtue of her having a new male heart. Although one of our patients wrote a book about this phenomenon—this cultured, artistic woman found herself suddenly drawn to chugging beers and riding motorcycles—medical science has not borne out such reports.

Women have a slightly higher likelihood of suffering some

rejection episodes after transplantation. This is likely a reflection of their exposure to a variety of antigens (immune proteins) from other individuals (their fetuses) during pregnancy, leading women to develop more antibodies (immune fighters). Most transplant patients have some episodes of rejection, but this slightly higher tendency among women does not impact their overall post-transplant survival. It used to be that the steroid medications used to prevent rejection after transplantation contributed to osteoporosis in women, but this is less common now, as most modern antirejection regimens limit or eliminate steroid medications after a few months.

## 6. THE ARTIFICIAL HEART

Artificial hearts have been used in humans since the 1960s. The Jarvik heart was tried in the early 1980s, replacing both the right and left sides of the heart. But—and this is a very important point— in the vast majority of patients, it is probably not necessary to replace both sides of the heart. As we discussed, most diseases affect predominantly the left side of the heart, which needs to be very powerful. On the other hand, the right side pumps only to the lungs and thus does not need to be nearly as strong.

Since the time of the original Jarvik heart, research has focused mainly on replacing the left side of the heart alone. Two companies have developed left side–only artificial heart devices: Novacor and HeartMate. After nearly twenty years of clinical experience, both have been FDA approved. They are like Ford and Chevy in that each has its supporters. HeartMate is a little less prone to clots and strokes, while Novacor (now called the WorldHeart) is a little more reliable.

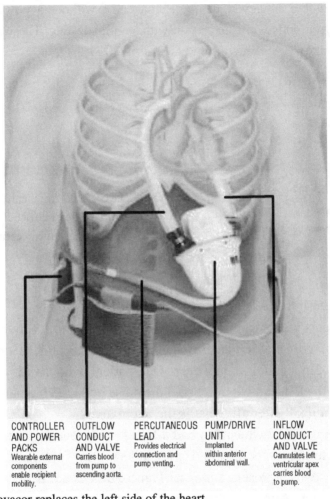

| CONTROLLER AND POWER PACKS | OUTFLOW CONDUCT AND VALVE | PERCUTANEOUS LEAD | PUMP/DRIVE UNIT | INFLOW CONDUCT AND VALVE |
|---|---|---|---|---|
| Wearable external components enable recipient mobility. | Carries blood from pump to ascending aorta. | Provides electrical connection and pump venting. | Implanted within anterior abdominal wall. | Cannulates left ventricular apex carries blood to pump. |

The Novacor replaces the left side of the heart.

Both Novacor and WorldHeart have a power cord that comes out through the skin and attaches to a power pack roughly the size of a portable CD player. Still, these patients can be very active, and Novacor especially can last a long, long time.

At present, patients unlikely to survive many months on the waiting list for a heart transplant are considered for an artificial heart. Patients too old for transplantation are eligible for an artificial heart device as well.

A number of newer devices, smaller or without a power cord exiting your body wall, are currently undergoing testing. These include the DeBakey/NASA device and the Jarvik 2000.

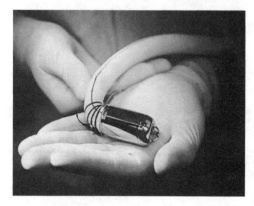

Jarvik 2000 "miniature" artificial heart device. Image © Jarvik Heart, Inc. Reprinted with permission.

These models may come into wider clinical use in the next several years if early beneficial data is confirmed more widely.

Patients with artificial heart devices can lead a full, active life—working, going to college, engaging in sports, and so on. The devices can be noisy, however. Our patient who lived with an implant the longest, when asked if the noise bothered him answered with a smile: "After all, what is the alternative?"

The AbioCor, which has had a lot of press recently, represents another foray into complete (right and left) heart replacement. The AbioCor does represent a major advance: it does not have a power cord. Rather, energy is transmitted by radio frequency from a battery pack worn about the waist. Now, radio frequency technology for energy transmission for medical purposes originated at our own institution some thirty years ago, by pioneer William W. L. Glenn for diaphragm pacing. AbioCor quite appropriately applied this same technology to the artificial heart. This mode of energy transmission represents a major advantage, because the skin barrier does not need to be pierced by a power cord, thus dramatically lessening the risk of long-term infection.

You can definitely feel the artificial heart beating inside you. Both the bulk of the device, usually placed in the belly, and the jolt of contraction are very obvious—as is the mechanical noise. In a movie theater, one of our patients was asked by another patron, "Can't you turn that noisy thing off?" His answer was a simple no.

With the artificial heart in place, the symptoms and limitations of the heart failure that the recipient previously suffered—such as fluid accumulation, shortness of breath, and lack of energy—literally vanish.

It's important to remember that since women are physically smaller, some of the devices, such as the Novacor and the Heart-Mate, can be difficult to fit in the body.

Whatever your cardiac ailment, whether coronary artery disease, valvular disease, arrhythmias, or heart failure, there is a procedure or an operation available that is highly likely to improve the quality and duration of your life. Many of these interventions represent the culmination of decades of surgical and technological innovation and refinement.

# 12

# GENETICS AND THE FEMALE HEART: WHAT YOU SHOULD KNOW ABOUT YOUR GENETIC LEGACY

## 1. CASE VIGNETTE: THREE GENERATIONS OF AORTIC DISSECTION

Mrs. Marshall had presented to the hospital in what is medically called *extremis*—that is, her condition was one of extreme jeopardy to life. Her aortic wall had split into layers, with the bloodstream forcing its way between the inner and outer layers. This is arguably the most severe condition that can afflict the human heart. Her split aorta had also ruptured, causing internal bleeding and compressing of the heart chambers themselves. Her blood pressure was vanishingly low. She was in a state of cardiogenic shock (inadequate flow due to heart impairment).

We took her to the operating room immediately—stat, as it is called on television and in real-life medical circumstances. We replaced her aorta. And she survived.

She was improving daily. About four days after her operation, as I was making rounds with my team, Mrs. Marshall was now well enough to have a conversation. I asked if any of her family members had ever had a problem similar to hers, an aortic dissection.

"Doctor," she said, "Don't you remember? You did the same operation for the same condition on my mother—two years ago."

Of course, I did not have any independent recollection, as such operations are very common on our service.

I asked whether any other family members had ever been affected. That's when Mrs. Marshall's tears began to well; they flowed incessantly. She composed herself only with difficulty.

She was finally able to tell me, "Doctor. My little girl. She died here at Yale New Haven Hospital. She was only ten. They told me it was something with her heart."

When we looked up the file, we found that the little girl had indeed died from aortic dissection—the youngest patient ever so afflicted at our institution.

So in the Marshall family, three generations were affected by this severe cardiac condition—acute aortic dissection.

This family history motivated us to investigate a possible hereditary nature of aortic aneurysm and dissection. Our investigations confirmed a strong genetic tendency. This recognition has the potential to save many lives.

## 2. CASE VIGNETTE: ANOTHER FAMILY WITH AORTIC DISSECTION

Just as I am writing this chapter on hereditary cardiac conditions, I have received a moving letter from Mrs. Cappiello, who is thanking me for saving her life. She underwent an operation to remove her aneurysm to prevent aortic dissection. She tells me that she is perfectly well now, some three years after her surgery. Next, she thanks me for bringing her family together to have them all checked. My team performed echo exams on about fifteen family members on Thanksgiving day—at their home, no less. (We find holidays a convenient time to study many family members.)

Then, the letter takes a different, sad tone. "Doctor," Mrs. Cappiello tells me, "My granddaughter Catherine did not come to that Thanksgiving dinner. She knew your team would be there, but she did not feel it was important enough to travel to Connecticut. I am writing to let you know that last week, in Cincinnati, she was rushed to the emergency room in full cardiac arrest. She was thirty-two. She did not survive. The autopsy found a ruptured aortic dissection. I am sharing this information with you so that you can amend your records to indicate yet another one of my family members affected."

Mrs. Cappiello went on to wonder whether her granddaughter might still be alive if she had just attended that Thanksgiving family screening. Mrs. Cappiello expressed appreciation for our scientific investigations into the hereditary nature of cardiac diseases, and aortic dissection in particular.

## 3. THE IMPORTANCE OF HEREDITY

You likely noticed that we have often mentioned hereditary tendencies in various diseases. The two case histories given at the beginning of this chapter illustrate the hereditary nature of cardiac disease vividly and unfortunately sadly.

For many decades, medical science has been able to draw conclusions that specific diseases are inherited from parents. Now, however, we find ourselves in an era in which the exact genetic mutations (changes, or abnormalities) that account for the hereditary nature of a disease are being pinpointed by detailed molecular genetic analysis.

We will illustrate this using our own Yale data on aortic aneurysm and dissection. Spurred by case histories like those that you read at the beginning of this chapter, we conducted hundreds upon hundreds of family interviews, aimed at completing what is called a family pedigree. In such a pedigree, each individual is represented by a circle (for females) or a square (for males). An open circle or square indicates an individual without the disease in question. A black circle or square indicates that the individual represented is affected by the disease being studied. An oblique line (cross-hatch) through the circle or square indicates a deceased individual.

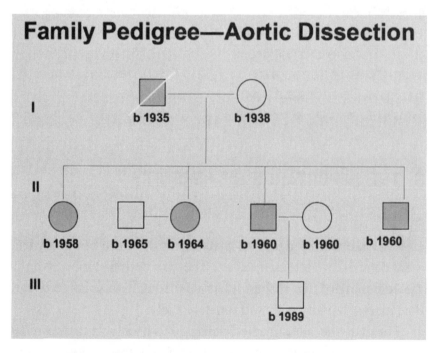

**Family Pedigree—Aortic Dissection**

Diagram courtesy of author.

The construction of these purely clinical charts allows medical scientists to characterize the clinical genetics of a disease. For example, in the case of aneurysm and dissection, we found that this disease usually follows a dominant pattern, being passed on if even a single parent is affected. Other diseases may be recessive, requiring that both parents be affected (a very uncommon circumstance) in order for the offspring to be affected. Many cardiac diseases have been characterized in this way.

The next step is to determine the specific chromosome (of the forty-six in human cells) affected by a particular disease. This is often done by linkage analysis, in which the errant chromosome is identified by its proximity to known chromosome markers. This technique provides a rough guide as to the location of the abnormal gene that causes a specific disease. This information is available for many human diseases. For example, in Marfan's syndrome, one cause of aneurysms, it is known that chromosome 15 is affected.

The final step is to identify the exact mutation (abnormality) in the genetic code that accounts for a specific disease; this is done by mapping each bit of information in the genetic code, using sophisticated techniques. For Marfan's syndrome, for example, over eighty specific mutations in the abnormal gene have been identified.

The genetic clarification of diseases—and cardiac disease in particular—represents a fundamental achievement in our understanding of the human body and its abnormalities. This promises to advance medicine to a level of sophistication never before accomplished or even contemplated in the history of humankind.

The following table below gives a broad overview of cardiac diseases that are now known to be hereditary, at least in part.

| DISEASE | HEREDITARY NATURE |
|---|---|
| Coronary artery disease | Heavily hereditary |
| Cardiomyopathy | Susceptibility to viral cardiomyopathy (muscle weakness) seems to be inherited. Hypertrophic cardiomyopathy (muscle weakness) heavily hereditary (over 100 mutations identified). |
| Aortic aneurysm and dissection | Heavily hereditary (mutations beginning to be identified). |
| Valvular heart disease | Mitral valve prolapse can be familial. |
| Stroke | Strongly hereditary. |
| Hypertension | Strongly hereditary. |

These genetic cardiac abnormalities include not only aneurysm disease but also coronary artery disease, arteriosclerosis in general, cardiomyopathy, valvular heart disease, stroke, and hypertension, among others.

As well, other specific disorders of the pumping strength of the heart, of the electrical conduction within the heart, and of the anatomic structure of the heart have been found to run in families. Many forms of congenital heart disease (in which there are "holes in the heart" or an abnormal size, shape, configuration, or connection of the heart valves and chambers) are highly genetic in their causation.

In arteriosclerosis and coronary artery disease, for example, a substance called Apolipoprotein E has been implicated. This substance, normally found in our bodies, is responsible for clearing excess cholesterol from our bloodstreams by delivering it to the liver, where it is detoxified. It is now known that many individuals with abnormally severe arteriosclerosis have genetically abnormal versions of Apolipoprotein E, so that the cholesterol is not adequately delivered to the liver for processing.[1] This abnormality may someday in the not-too-distant future be treated by gene therapy.

We do not want you to feel inferior or responsible because you have heart disease and you may pass on (or already have passed on) this same tendency to your children. We are all dealt a genetic hand of cards. One of the wonders of nature is that we are all different, each of us with inherent strengths and weaknesses. We each have genes that are better than average and genes that are poorer than average. We encourage you to focus on the positives in your genetic legacy.

Please keep in mind that, although we may now recognize the genetic component of many, many heart problems, we are on the verge of being able to treat, or even cure, these diseases by virtue of the advances in understanding at the fundamental molecular genetic level. There is every possibility that we will soon be able to replace the abnormal genes with normal ones—thus thwarting the disease before it can manifest as any abnormality in the structure of the heart. This is the dawn of a new era of understanding of human disease, heart disease included. The genetic understanding will help us with early diagnosis, with design of conventional drugs and, ultimately, with gene repair.[2]

Until genetic therapy is realized, I have one specific instruction for you upon completing your reading of this book: "Pick the right Parents."

# Chapter
# 13
# LIVING WITH HEART DISEASE

**W**e hope that this book will help you regardless of the state of your heart disease. If you do not have heart disease, we hope that this book can help you prevent it. If you do have heart disease, we hope that this book can help you keep it from worsening. Regardless of the state of advancement of your disease, medical science has treatments that can be applied, be they medications, catheterization lab interventions, surgical procedures, or even cardiac transplantation, the artificial heart, or experimental therapies.

## 1. KNOWING YOUR OPTIONS

- *Heart disease in a family member.* Many of you have relatives with heart disease. If so, the information in this book will help you guide the women in your family through the process of diagnosis and treatment. (Of course, this is in correlation with consulting with a physician.)
- *Free of disease.* You may have no evidence of heart disease at this point. We hope that many of you are in this category. If so, the information in this book can help you recognize the symptoms of heart disease in women you know and in yourself, if and when they should appear. The preventive strategies in this book can also help you remain "free of disease."

- *High risk factors.* Some of you may have no evidence of heart disease but harbor known risk factors, such as a strong family history, high cholesterol, high blood pressure, diabetes, obesity, smoking, or a sedentary lifestyle. The information in this book will help you delay or avoid heart disease as long as possible.

- *Known heart disease.* Some of you will have known heart disease—perhaps coronary artery disease, valvular heart disease, congestive heart failure, or arrhythmias. The information throughout this book will help to guide you through the maze of options for diagnosis and treatment. In this chapter, we wish to focus further on those of you in this group, with active heart disease. We wish to share some advice on coping with this diagnosis.

## 2. ACCEPTING THE DIAGNOSIS

We can tell you—from years of experience in caring for thousands of patients—that each and every human being will develop some type of illness during his or her lifespan. For you, it happens to be heart disease. Each of us gets positive and negative genetic tendencies from our parents. You may have inherited your tendency to heart disease. We are sure that, simultaneously, you inherited many strengths, both physical and mental. Please be assured, as you have seen in the preceeding pages, that many, if not most, forms of heart disease are eminently treatable—with medications or surgery. We suggest accepting the diagnosis, without despondency, and instead focusing your efforts on obtaining the optimal assessments and treatments. Our desire is that this book will help you maintain and interpret the information and advice given by your physicians.

# 3. SUPPORT FROM FAMILY MEMBERS

None of us can be an island, isolated from the help and support of others. Be sure to have a loved one or friend with you when you go for your doctor's visits, helping you interpret and remember the information provided. As we have seen many times, the support and love from your family and friends can indeed help you through the difficulty of a cardiac illness.

# 4. LIFESTYLE MODIFICATIONS

## Diet

There are many useful books written on dieting. The fact is that we don't really know which diets are the best. Diets and recommendations go in cycles and pass through fads. We will emphasize a few uncontested facts, however.

### Salt

Patients with high blood pressure should use salt sparingly, but most patients with coronary artery disease do not have to be particularly concerned about their salt intake. If, however, the patient with coronary artery disease has congestive heart failure, then salt restriction is necessary.

### Body Mass Index

Body mass index (BMI) compares your weight to your height. Of course, taller individuals should weigh more, and BMI takes that relationship into account. You can calculate your body mass index by dividing your weight in pounds by your height (squared) in inches, with the conversion factor shown in the equation below:

$$\text{Body Mass Index (BMI)} = 703 \times \frac{\text{weight (pounds)}}{\text{height (inches)}^2}$$

You should aim to get your own body mass index into the range of 25 to 26. Of course, as we approach or exceed middle age, some increase in weight is almost inevitable, so a measure of leniency in expected BMI is warranted. A dangerous BMI would be 30 or above.

## Blood Pressure

Elevated blood pressure is a prime factor in bringing on arteriosclerosis, so controlling your blood pressure is one of the most crucial steps you can take to prevent or slow the disease's progress

Lifestyle changes are important in controlling blood pressure, and you can do a lot to bring blood pressure down to normal. These lifestyle changes relate to (1) moderation in the use of salt in foods, (2) achieving an optimal weight (a BMI of 25–26), and (3) a regular exercise program. To the extent that stress can be eliminated from the daily routine, that is desirable. These lifestyle changes are sometimes sufficient to control high blood pressure, but medication must at times be added to ensure a normal blood pressure around the clock.

## Cigarette Smoking

*Cigarette smoking is another prime factor in causing arteriosclerosis. Yes, you absolutely, positively need to stop smoking.* Smoking damages your arteries immensely, sending substances into your bloodstream that are like sandpaper scraping the inner lining (endothelium) of your arteries. Your chance of restoring cardiac health nearly vanishes—no matter what treatments, medications, or operations are applied—if you continue to smoke. Get help quitting from your general practitioner or internist. Many drugs, patches, and the like are available today to help you in your battle against cigarettes. Kick this habit that is literally killing you.

## Drinking

Believe it or not, alcohol in moderation is not bad for your heart. It does not contribute to arteriosclerosis. In fact, as many of you have heard, wine in small daily doses actually protects your arteries. Please keep in mind, however, that heavy consumption of alcohol, while it does not hurt your arteries, can result in direct damage to your heart muscle, the so-called alcoholic cardiomyopathy, not to mention the potential for damage to your liver.

## Exercise

Exercise is beneficial in a number of ways. The heart is a muscle and, like any other muscle in the body, becomes more efficient when used. A well-conditioned athlete generally has a slow heart rate, as her heart can pump more blood with each beat. Further, other muscles become more efficient with exercise and therefore extract oxygen more effectively from the blood. Therefore, the heart does not have to pump as much blood each minute. Exercise generally is useful in lowering blood pressure, by about 10 mmHg, as small blood vessels dilate or relax after the exercise is over. Ancillary benefits include the fact that exercise burns calories, is a useful adjunct to weight reduction, raises your level of HDL (the good cholesterol) by about 10 percent, and can relieve stress. If you are a diabetic, exercise will lower your blood glucose levels by using up sugar and by making your body more sensitive to its own insulin. An individual who exercises regularly will generally not be a smoker, thereby eradicating a potent risk factor to the development of coronary artery disease.

## Diabetes Control

If you are a diabetic, you must control your diabetes to prevent rapid progression of coronary artery disease and arteriosclerosis. Diabetes causes especially severe coronary artery disease, which tends to narrow the entire artery from top to bottom. For nondiabetics, the narrowings seem to be more localized. In diabetics, even the small branches are often diseased. This can make it difficult to find a spot to place a graft during the coronary artery bypass procedure. In diabetes, the arteries tend to be diseased from top to bottom, without even a soft spot conducive to touch-down of the bypass graft.

You can aim to keep your pre-prandial (before meals) blood sugars and your bedtime blood sugars around 100 mg/dl. This will mitigate the impact of diabetes on your blood vessels and organs.

## A Complete Set of Suggestions

Dr. Salim Yusuf at the McMaster University in Toronto has identified nine specific measures each patient with heart disease can take to improve her future.[1] These measures also make sense for those who do not have heart disease currently but are eager to prevent its development. The measures are linked directly to the nine most important risk factors leading to heart disease, which account for about 90 percent of the statistical risk for heart disease.

1. *Control your cholesterol.* We discussed the types of cholesterol and their importance earlier. As a start, you need to
know your cholesterol level. If it is high, you can use diet,
exercise, and drugs, if necessary, to bring a high cholesterol
into line.

2. *Diabetes.* You need to avoid diabetes. Diabetes dramatically
increases the frequency and severity of arteriosclerosis.
Keep your weight down as you get older; this will help
tremendously in avoiding late-onset diabetes. Regular exercise will help as well. If you already have diabetes, managing your sugar meticulously will help prevent arteriosclerosis.

3. *Control your stress.* Stress is an inherent part of life and definitely contributes to coronary artery disease. Although you
cannot eliminate stress from your life, you should take
measures to control or eliminate recurrent sources of severe
stress, interpersonal, familial, or job-related.

4. *Obesity.* Obesity adds dramatically to your risk of heart disease, as well as contributes to high blood pressure and diabetes. Interestingly, recent studies have shown that abdominal obesity—that around your belly—is most dangerous.
Maintaining a healthy weight will help tremendously in
keeping your heart and blood vessels healthy.

5. *Cigarette smoking.* Smoking cigarettes damages the lining
of your arteries, paving the way for cholesterol deposits to
form. You simply must stop smoking. There are many aids
for smoking cessation currently available through your pharmacy or general practitioner that can help you.

6. *High blood pressure.* High blood pressure damages your
blood vessels, which leads to arteriosclerosis and heart disease. Know your blood pressure. It is usually measured in
your doctor's office. You can also buy economical and accu-

rate automatic blood pressure monitors at your pharmacy. If your blood pressure is high, work with your doctor to bring it into line, through weight reduction, diet, or medications. Your heart will thank you.

7. *Alcohol.* A drink a day is actually *beneficial.* Can you believe that? We are actually recommending that you have a drink a day, as families do in Europe around the dinner table. Red wine is best, but other forms of alcohol are also helpful. We think this is because alcohol prevents platelets from becoming too sticky, which can clog small vessels. However, if you consume more than a drink or two per day, you may promote heart failure or as everyone knows, damage your liver.

8. *Exercise.* Exercise is beneficial in every conceivable way. Exercise helps to keep your weight in check, decreases the likelihood of diabetes, drops your blood pressure, and preserves your muscle mass. You should partake in aerobic exercise (even walking suffices) at least five days a week.

9. *Diet.* Fruits and vegetables are the nutritional keys to a healthy heart. They keep your cholesterol in check and cleanse damaging chemicals from around your cells.

We just wish you could follow step number ten as well—*choose your parents carefully*! Heredity is the other key factor in your developing heart disease, and a very potent contributor at that. However, since you cannot really choose your parents, you should concentrate on steps number one through nine.

# Chapter
# 14
# NINE MORE THINGS YOU NEED TO KNOW

**H**ere, we will review briefly a number of items in the form of questions we have actually received:

## 1. HOW ARE WOMEN PROTECTED FROM ARTERIOSCLEROSIS UNTIL MENOPAUSE?

To some extent, women are indeed protected against heart disease—especially the hardening of the arteries that affects men so commonly—from birth until menopause. It is extremely uncommon for a premenopausal woman to suffer from angina and experience a heart attack. In fact, the only women who fall prey to this disease early in life are generally those who have juvenile onset diabetes or familial hyperlipidemia (high lipid, or fat, levels in the blood). The abnormalities of the arteries are so profound in these diseases that even being a woman of child-bearing age cannot confer sufficient protection.

However, after menopause women catch up very quickly with men in the likelihood of acquiring coronary artery disease. Black women are especially prone to cardiovascular disease and heart-related death. In fact, heart disease is the number-one killer of women, outpacing even cancer. Moreover, while deaths from heart disease in men are decreasing, deaths from heart disease in women are actually *increasing*.

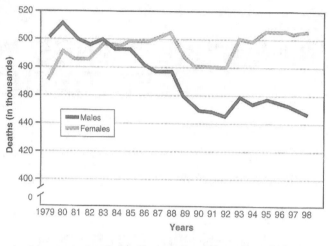

Reprinted with permission from the American Heart Association.

This is an epidemic that requires patient education, physician emphasis, and dedicated cardiovascular research.

Not only do women catch up with men quickly after menopause, but heart disease in women, when it occurs, is more virulent. As we have seen in other chapters, heart attacks and heart failure are more lethal in women than in men.

While astutely cognizant of breast and uterine cancer, many women are unaware of the critical toll exacted by coronary artery disease on womens' lives. So gender can confer protection, but only until about the early fifties, when menstruation ceases. It is important to recognize that even being a woman does not protect at all against other forms of heart disease besides arteriosclerosis, such as congenital heart disease or valvular heart disease.

Despite decades of concerted research, we still do not know how women are protected. There is a general consensus that the hormonal milieu—a woman's estrogen—somehow prevents arteriosclerotic deposits in the arteries of the heart. We simply do not know how or why this is so. In fact, tremendous attention has been directed toward determining if giving estrogen treatment can extend the hormonal benefits into later stages of a woman's life. The simple answer is no—hormone therapy after menopause does not protect against heart disease. In fact, for certain women, the risk of heart disease seems to increase somewhat. (See the chapter on hormone therapy.) A study conducted by the NIH was actually terminated early because women on hormone therapy did more poorly than those without. The Women's Health Initiative trial suggests that estrogen-progestin therapy will not prevent heart attacks. The study followed healthy postmenopausal women aged 50 to 79 years. Women taking estogen-progestin therapy had an increased risk of breast cancer, stroke, heart disease, and blood clots over an average follow-up of 5-years. Subsequent analysis suggests that the increased risk may be confined to older women, however further reseach is ongoing.

One theory as to how women are protected has to do with the body's iron stores. Iron is essential for our red blood cells, the ones that carry oxygen to all parts of our body. But it has been shown that iron contributes to arteriosclerosis. Because of menstrual flow, women generally have lower blood counts—fewer red blood cells and less iron in their bodies. Thus, it follows logically that men are at greater risk and that women lose their protection at menopause, when the monthly loss of iron ceases.

While in some ways an attractive concept, the iron hypothesis has never been proven conclusively.

## 2. HOW ABOUT THE "PILL"? IS IT REALLY AS BAD AS THEY SAY?

The vast majority of women can use the contraceptive pill without adverse consequences. There is no doubt, however, that the risk of cardiovascular problems is several-fold higher in women on the pill than in those who are not. Still, the likelihood of a problem occurring is on the order of one or two in ten thousand women on the pill.[1]

The problems that do occur tend to fall into two categories. First, women on the pill can manifest excess clotting in the veins, sometimes accompanied by passage of clots into the lungs. This usually occurs in the veins of the legs, where it is called deep vein thrombosis, or DVT. Second, women on the pill can develop accelerated arteriosclerosis.

The risk of problems from the pill is higher in women over thirty-five years of age, women who smoke, and, of course, diabetics and obese women. If you are a young, nonsmoking, trim, nondiabetic woman without prior thrombosis or heart disease, it is perfectly reasonable for you to consider using the pill for contraception.

## 3. I HEARD ON TV THAT MY MIGRAINES MIGHT BE CAUSED BY A HOLE IN MY HEART. HOW CAN THIS BE?

That is correct. This possibility is being considered.

Migraines are extremely common in women. It has very recently been noticed that women with migraine headaches commonly have a patent foramen ovale, which is Latin for "a small hole in the heart." It is a variant of atrial septal defect, which refers to a hole in the wall between the upper chambers of the heart, or atria. See figure 14.1.

We do not understand exactly how such a small opening results in a migraine. It is presumed that small clots, originating in the legs after sitting or standing for a long time, pass through the small hole to reach the brain. In the brain, these small clots may cause spasms of the brain arteries, leading to the pain and other phenomena (auras and the like), which are characteristic of migraines.

In fact, so strong is the interest in patent foramen ovale as a

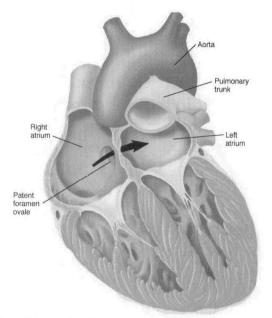

Figure 14.1. Atrial septal defect—a hole in the heart.

cause of migraines that a multicenter trial approved by the FDA has begun. In affected women, the hole is closed by a small device (called an umbrella because of its shape) passed through the veins, without an incision.

Within five to seven years, we should know if this form of treatment is truly effective for migraines, which burden and often incapacitate so many millions of women.

## 4. DOES A WOMAN NEED ANY SPECIAL WOUND CARE AFTER OPEN HEART SURGERY?

For extremely large-breasted women, the weight of the breasts themselves can pull against the median sternotomy incision (vertical incision over the breastbone). Wearing a brassiere, even in the ICU, can help alleviate the skin tension and the accompanying discomfort.

The so-called intertriginous folds—those areas under the breast where the breast tissue rubs against the skin of the chest—can be a source of problems. Moisture and excoriation in this region can lead to infection, even of the chest wound itself. It is essential to maintain good hygiene in this region before operation and to keep this area clean and dry after surgery. Sometimes a small surgical dressing under each breast can assist in prevent the rubbing of the skin and excoriation.

## 5. I DON'T WANT THE INCISION DOWN THE MIDDLE OF MY CHEST. WHAT ALTERNATIVES DO I HAVE?

This question comes up most often among young women or women who have not married and had their children, as well as others. This is understandable. These women may be having surgery for congenital heart disease or for valvular heart disease. In a bathing suit or in a shirt with an open collar, the incision can show. Many women are also concerned about what a significant other may think.

For some young women, and others with these concerns, we use a submammary incision. This incision hides in the creases under the breasts. See figure 14.2.

With this alternate incision, the scar hides in the crease under each breast, leading to improved cosmetics and avoiding the up-and-down traditional incision. It is hardly visible, even when the woman is naked. With such a horizontal incision, we can still open the breastbone vertically, up and down. While the submammary approach adds somewhat to the complexity of the operation, this is usually not a serious factor.

If you are concerned about a vertical scar, ask your surgeon about the submammary approach or other incisions that may be

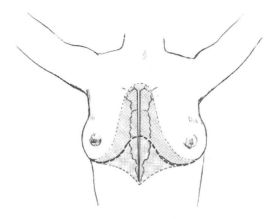

Figure 14.2. The submammary incision.

useful in your particular situation. Mitral valve surgery, for example, can be performed through a small incision confined to the region under your right breast.

Nothing is free in life, however. The submammary approach, or other alternate incisions, share the drawback that they can produce numbness in the nipple area. While this is often temporary, that is not always the case, and you should be aware of this possibility.

## 6. WHAT ARE THE DANGERS OF PREGNANCY ON THE HEART?

Pregnancy most definitely has a major impact on the heart. As noted earlier, the woman's circulatory system, by the end of pregnancy, is responsible for supplying blood and oxygen to a growing, newly developing human being in her womb. The heart also needs to supply the greater body mass of the woman herself that comes about during the course of pregnancy. The amount of circulating blood nearly doubles by the end of pregnancy, so the workload of the heart is doubled. The blood flow to the uterus increases from a trickle to more than a quart per minute. The blood flow to the breasts increases. The blood flow to the skin increases by half again above normal, possibly as a means of dissipating heat. This situation strains a normal heart, let alone a diseased heart. If a woman has underlying heart disease, usually of the valves, the heart may strain or fail during pregnancy. Fortunately, this scenario does not arise frequently. The high blood pressure that is common in the last trimester of pregnancy also puts an additional burden on the heart. The circulatory changes that accompany pregnancy are depicted in figure 1.3 (page 34).

If you know you have heart disease, you need to be monitored during your pregnancy not only by your gynecologist, but also by a cardiologist. Sometimes you do not know you have heart disease until the extra burden of pregnancy unmasks cardiac symptoms.

The testing of your heart is somewhat limited in pregnancy because of the fetus. We never wish to expose the fetus to the potential damaging influence of x-rays. Echocardiograms, however, are entirely safe. In fact, your baby has many echo exams through your abdominal wall even during a normal pregnancy.

## Pregnancy and Coumadin

Some young women do require an artificial heart valve and need to be treated with Coumadin. At times, these women have not completed their child-bearing and want to become pregnant despite the artificial heart valve and the Coumadin treatment. This is somewhat difficult, but definitely possible and reasonably safe.

First off, Coumadin itself is not safe for the baby and results in a high rate of miscarriage. Coumadin is what we call teratogenic, or damaging to the fetus—in fact, highly so. It is simply not appropriate to take Coumadin during your pregnancy, especially in the

earlier phases. (Very recently this dogma has been being ques-
tioned, and Coumadin may soon be permited in selected cases.)

So adjustments need to be made. Some women can be carried
through pregnancy without Coumadin, often with aspirin alone.
More commonly, we substitute the drug heparin for Coumadin.
Heparin is not teratogenic. Heparin and heparinlike drugs do not
cross the placenta, so the fetus is not directly exposed to them. The
problem is that heparin cannot be taken orally and is given by subcutaneous injection, just as diabetics inject their insulin. This is not
too onerous once you are used to it. An alternate form of heparin,
known as Lovenox, can be given at more widely spaced intervals,
so you should not need to give yourself a shot more than once, or
at most twice, a day.

This whole process is safer if your artificial valve is in the aortic
position, where it is relatively less prone to clots. If your valve is in
the mitral position, the risk of forming clots on the valve is a bit
higher. Still, with careful coordination between your obstetrician
and your cardiologist, and a large measure of patience on your part,
you can be carried through your pregnancy. The effort will all be
worthwhile when your new baby is placed on your lap after
delivery.

Because of these issues related to Coumadin, many young
women opt for biological valves instead of mechanical valves. (See
chapter 11, which covers open-heart surgery.) Biological valves do
not require blood thinners, and these Coumadin–pregnancy issues
become obviated. However, the biological valve will wear out after
about fifteen years, and another operation will be necessary.

Two very serious specific cardiac conditions can affect a
woman during pregnancy and, though rare, deserve mention. These
are discussed below.

# 7. WHAT IS PERI-PARTUM CARDIOMYOPATHY?

### Case Vignette: Peri-Partum Cardiomyopathy

I will never forget walking into this patient's room in the coronary care unit. After some ten thousand patients I've operated on, it takes a very special case to remain clearly in my memory—and Lauren's case was indeed special and touching. Lauren had given birth to her baby boy; the obstetrician had just started to put the baby in Loren's lap; and, just then, Lauren suffered cardiac arrest. She lapsed into cardiogenic shock (inadequate forward pumping of blood by the heart) from peri-partum cardiomyopathy (weakness of the heart muscle brought on by pregnancy and delivery). Lauren had been maintained on a breathing tube and machine, on powerful IV drugs to stimulate the heart, and on a mechanical support device called an intra-aortic balloon pump. She had been sedated and paralyzed for the entire month. She had never seen her baby. The baby had never felt its mother's touch. And, at this point, it was looking doubtful that either would happen, as Lauren's chances of recovery appeared extremely poor.

I had been called to see Lauren to consider placing her on an artificial heart device, as her heart was failing progressively, and the balloon pump was no longer sufficient.

We did so. Lauren survived the operation. With the artificial heart, she lived long enough for a donor heart to become available and, ultimately, we replaced Lauren's failed heart with a strong, reliable donor heart. She saw her baby. Her baby felt her mother's touch and her love.

That was seven years ago.

Lauren just sent me a card with a picture of herself and her baby daughter.

Lauren had almost suc-cumbed to the unusual, but potentially devastating, condition known as peri-partum cardiomyopathy.

Very rarely, for reasons that are not entirely clear, a woman can develop a very weak heart around the end of her pregnancy or shortly after delivery. The ejection fraction (pumping strength of the heart) may fall dramatically. This phenomenon is called peri-partum cardiomyopathy. "Peri-" means "around the time of"; "partum" means "delivery"; and "cardiomyopathy" means "weakness of the heart." Fortunately, peri-partum cardiomyopathy is seen only about once in several thousand pregnancies. African American women, older pregnant women, women carrying twins, and women who have had multiple prior deliveries are a bit more prone to this disease.[2] Peri-partum cardiomyopathy may be extremely severe at times. The woman may even lapse into shock. She may require an artificial heart or a heart transplant. If these advanced measures are not available, peri-partum cardiomyopathy can be lethal in up to one-half of cases. In others, the syndrome is mild or even self-limited, with return to normal function over weeks to months. We do not know what causes this disease, in exactly whom to suspect that it may occur, or how to prevent it.

## 8. WHAT IS PERI-PARTUM AORTIC DISSECTION?

One other very special and severe cardiac condition can occur during pregnancy—aortic dissection. This is a tearing of the internal layers of the aorta brought on by the added circulatory burden of advanced pregnancy, by the high blood pressure of late pregnancy, and especially by the dramatic straining and bearing down needed for childbirth. Most women affected by this very serious condition are made vulnerable by an underlying aortic enlargement or weakening. If you have a history of aneurysms or dissections in your family, please bring this to the attention of your gynecologist. Special precautions need to be taken. Fortunately, peri-partum aortic dissection is rare. When it does occur, it threatens both the mother and the baby.

# 9. HOW DOES HEART DISEASE AFFECT SEXUALITY IN WOMEN?

There is emerging scientific information to corroborate the general sense that a vigorous sex life is conducive to cardiovascular health in women. One study found that a measure of cardiovascular health called heart rate variability was improved in women who had regular sex with a partner.[4]

## How About Sex after Bouts of Heart Disease?

There is no question that the medical profession has been inadequate in explaining to women the important fact that cardiac disease need not imply an end to their sexual lives and fulfillment. Perhaps due to discomfort with the subject or a sense that issues of survival take precedence, doctors avoid conversations about sexuality with their recovering heart patients.

In fact, not only is it possible for you to resume sexual activity after a cardiac event, but such resumption is an important step in achieving the emotional fulfillment that is vital to cardiac health.

A recent study in Spain found that "sexual activity was practically non-existent in the women surveyed" after cardiac events.[4]

This needn't be so. Whether you have had a heart attack or heart failure, or even an artificial heart or a heart transplant, you can, and indeed should, resume sexual activity. We usually recommend resuming gradually about ten to fourteen days after your discharge from the hospital after a cardiac event or procedure (such as a heart attack, an angioplasty, a pacemaker or a defibrillator, or an open-heart operation).

It has been estimated that the exertion level of sexual activity is roughly equivalent to that of walking briskly up two flights of stairs.[5] In general, the average maximal heart rate with peak sexual activity is approximately 120 beats per minute (less if you are taking medications such as betablockers), and this will last for less than three minutes. Some people, based on news reports or hearsay, fear that a heart attack may occur during sex. This is actually a vanishingly rare phenomenon—on the order of one in hundreds of thousands of sexual encounters. There are only very few categories of uncontrolled heart disease—such as extreme high blood pressure, unstable angina, a very recent heart attack, very poor heart function (ejection fraction), severe arrhythmias, or severe, uncorrected valvular heart disease—in which there may be substantial risk from sexual activity.[6] Even in such circumstances, your doctor can usually improve your cardiac situation adequately to permit sexual activity. Be sure to ask your cardiologist about his recommendations regarding sexual activity.

Please keep in mind that your medications may influence your desire for sex and your physiologic response. Many women with heart disease report difficulties in sexual activity.[7] This is an important part of your well-being, so please let your doctor know if you are having problems. Chances are that a medication adjustment or alteration may be beneficial.

In addition, patients often have symptoms of depression after a cardiac event that can markedly reduce sexual interest and capacity.

These symptoms are not unexpected and in the majority of cases go away within a few months. Social support and participation in cardiac rehabilitation has been shown to decrease symptoms of depression in women with heart disease. If you continue to have depression, speak with your physician, as it may lead to sexual problems with your significant other.

It is also quite possible that your husband has heart disease as well, and you may be concerned for his well-being during sexual activity. This may be a major factor in interfering with sexual activity after your own bout with heart disease.[8] Please be reassured that, for your husband as well as yourself, it is very likely that a return to an active and safe sexual life should be feasible. Do not let fear get in the way of a fulfilling relationship.

Here are some suggestions on how to restart your intimate relationship:

- Pick a good time of the day for both you and your partner. Both of you should be relaxed and well rested. Have open discussions about restarting sexual activities because you both may have anxieties!
- Warm up as you would before any physical activity! Foreplay will raise the heart rate and blood pressure slowly.
- Sex positions using the arms to support the body require more work, so avoid these for a couple of months.
- If you have trouble getting back to a sexual routine, start slower by perhaps just holding your partner and initially limiting activity to foreplay.
- Talk to you partner: this involves a couple, not just an individual. Anxiety will put more work on the heart and make it harder for you to return to your normal sexual life.
- Women should discuss with their doctor any chest pain experienced during sexual intercourse. Nitroglycerine, a medica-

tion that dilates the blood vessels to the heart, may be prescribed. (Never share medications! If your male partner uses Viagra, a highly effective medication to treat erectile dysfunction, you should never give him your nitroglycerin. Men who are using nitroglycerin pills or patches, or who need to use nitroglycerin by spray or pills under the tongue to relieve angina, should not use Viagra. Viagra and nitroglycerin taken together may cause significant and severe drops in blood pressure.)

- Problems with sexual desire and/or function should always be discussed with your physician. A change in sexual desire and/or performance could be related to your medications. However, never discontinue medications without discussing with your doctor.

The bottom line is that we want you to enjoy a fulfilling sex life, and this is very possible, despite the fact that you have had some cardiac problems or interventions.

# Chapter
# 15
# PROSPECTS FOR THE FUTURE

**M**edical science had made tremendous advances in heart care in the last half of the twentieth century. But the prospects for the twenty-first century are nothing short of extraordinary.

First of all, in the last decade or so, we have come to understand very clearly that, in terms of heart disease, women are not just small men. They have different symptoms and manifest different patterns of heart disease. Much of this book has focused specifically on such differences. There is every likelihood that these differences will continue to be explored and better understood in the coming years.

Cardiac diagnosis is improving by leaps and bounds. Imaging of the heart by computerized equipment has given us previously unparalleled precision in visualizing coronary arteries and cardiac valves and chambers. There is every evidence that we are just scratching the surface of what imaging can and will do.

Medical therapies improve every year. We have better and better drugs for cholesterol control, for heart failure, for arrhythmias, and for angina. The future holds the prospect for "personalized" medications based on a particular patient's profile. It is no longer a situation of "one drug fits all." An important aspect of personalization will take into account the patient's gender.

Surgical treatments have shown to advance regularly and powerfully. The years ahead are likely to see major advances in control of rejection in heart transplantation and in artificial heart technology.

Increased understanding of the genetic underpinnings of heart diseases, made possible by the recently completed mapping of the human genome, raises the distinct possibility that heart diseases will be treated by directed gene therapy in the future.

Women can take heart that as they age their own cardiac disease will be diagnosed and treated better than ever before. They can also take solace in knowing that heart disease in their daughters (and sons) will be diagnosed and treated better than ever before—and, we hope, ultimately be prevented before it even occurs.

In the meantime, you can seize the moment to know as much as you can about your own health and the state of your heart, and—as we have seen in this book—you can take steps to improve your life and your future.

# Appendix

## INCREASE YOUR STRENGTH AND STAY HEALTHY

### BASIC STRENGTH PROGRAM GUIDELINES:

Strength training is an important part of a health and fitness program. We lose approximately 30 percent of our muscle tissue and 50 percent of our strength between the ages of fifty and eighty if we do not perform regular strength-promoting activities. Since the amount of muscle tissue a person has is directly related to how many calories she burns, the loss of muscles with age results in a lower metabolic rate. Thus a gradual increase in body fat is likely over time. In addition, the loss of strength makes it more difficult to perform everyday activities, leading to fatigue and, in some cases, even a loss of independence. A well-balanced strength-training program can prevent, slow, or reverse these losses. It improves strength for everyday activities, bone and joint health, posture, and endurance as well as helps maintain or increase metabolism to help control weight.

♥   ♥   ♥

The appendix and all photos are from the McConnel Heart Health Center, courtesy of Teresa Caulin-Glaser, MD, Executive Director.

# A strength-training program has the following components:

♥ **Frequency:** two to three nonconsecutive days per week is recommended.

♥ **Intensity:** The difficulty level should be from somewhat hard to hard for the last few repetitions of each exercise to be most effective. It is imperative to use correct form (described below) for every repetition to get the best results and to protect yourself from possible injury.

♥ **Type:** Resistance bands, weight machines, free weights, and/or group exercise classes in water or on land are all effective strength training options.

♥ **Time:** The amount of time you spend on resistance training will depend on your individual goals and interests; however, an effective resistance-training program can typically be completed in thirty minutes or less.

♥ **Progression:** Increasing the resistance will lead to increases in strength. Add a small amount of weight when you reach the top number of recommended repetitions (generally twelve or fifteen) in consecutive workouts. Be sure to perform the minimum number of repetitions (generally eight or ten) on the first workout with the new weight. Take several workouts to work up to the top number of repetitions again, then repeat the cycle. Do not sacrifice good form to increase your weight.

♥ **Warm up and cool down:** Begin and end your routine with five or more minutes of light aerobic activity followed by stretching. This helps your body transition from your everyday activities to your exercise routine by redirecting blood flow and lubricating joints.

# Correct form consists of:

♥ **Controlled speed:** Generally, two to four seconds is recommended, in each direction of the movement, when beginning a strength- training program. This assures that your muscles are doing the work and you are not using momentum or gravity to move the weight.

♥ **Proper range of motion:** Move through the full and natural range of movement while protecting the joints at both ends of the movement. This assures that you work the muscles so they get stronger while you protect the joints and connective tissue from excessive stress, weight-bearing, and possible injury.

♥ **Normal breathing:** Maintain an open airway by breathing normally during weight lifting. Also, avoid excessive squeezing of the handgrips. This will help avoid large increases in blood pressure that can occur when holding your breath and gripping tightly while pushing or pulling a load.

♥ **Proper posture:** A tall, elongated spine, with your chest lifted, provides a strong position and decreases compression on the intervertebral discs. If necessary, a towel roll is an ideal support for the natural arch in your low back on appropriate exercises. Look straight ahead to keep the cervical spine properly aligned.

Many of the following illustrations are shown with resistance bands. You can substitute dumbells for the resistance bands, if you wish.

# Squats

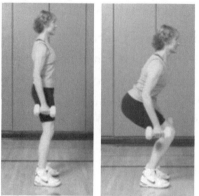

1. Stand upright with your feet shoulder-width apart, your knees slightly bent, and a dumbell in each hand at your sides.
2. Bend your knees and hips, keeping your back straight and your head up and your eyes looking forward. Be sure to keep some of your weight back on your heels, keeping your knees from going forward past your toes. Lower your body to a position slightly higher than sitting in a chair, while maintaining correct posture.
3. Slowly return to the starting position and repeat ten to fifteen times.

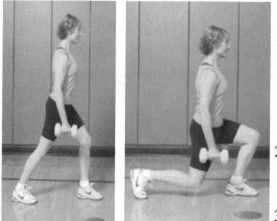

# Lunges

1. Stand upright with your feet shoulder-width apart holding a dumbell in each hand.
2. Step backward with your right foot.
3. Bend your knees, lowering your body to a position slightly higher than sitting in a chair. Be sure to keep your left knee from going forward past your toes.
4. Return the left foot to starting position. Repeat ten to twelve times for each leg.

# Single-Leg Calf Raise

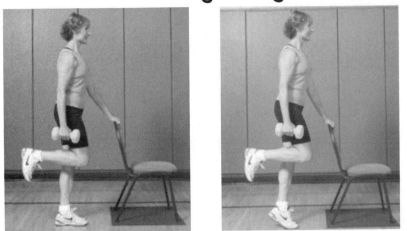

1. Stand on your right foot with a dumbbell in your left hand, placing your right hand against a wall or the back of a chair for balance.
2. Extend your ankle, raising up on your toes.
3. Slowly lower to the starting position and repeat ten to fifteen times. Repeat on the opposite side.

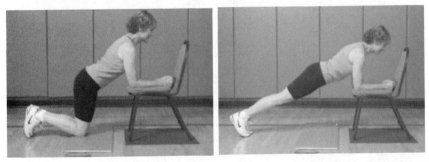

# Forearm Plank

1. Start with your forearms on a chair or on the floor and your knees on the floor.
2. Lift your knees off the floor simultaneously to a position in which your body is in a straight line.
3. Keep your body straight. Set a goal of holding this position for thirty to sixty seconds.

# Seated Row

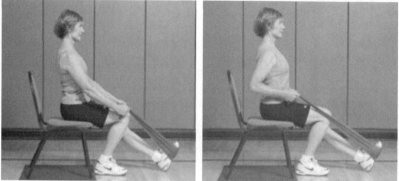

1. Sit upright in a chair with one leg extended. Wrap the middle of the resistance band under your foot and hold one end in each hand.
2. Start with your arms extended toward your foot. In a controlled motion, push your elbows back while lifting your chest.
3. Slowly return to the starting position and repeat ten to fifteen times.

# Chest Press

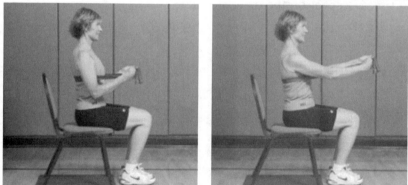

1. Sit upright in a chair with a resistance band behind your back and under each arm. Place one end of the resistance band in each hand. Bend your elbows to about 90 degrees and keep your hands about chest height.
2. In a controlled motion, move your hands forward until your elbows are just slightly bent.
3. Slowly return to the starting position and repeat ten to fifteen times.

# Resistance Band Squats

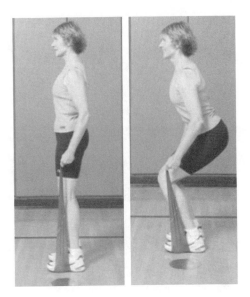

1. Start with the middle of a resistance band under both feet. Stand with your feet shoulder-width apart and your knees slightly bent. Keep your hands at your sides, with one end of the resistance band in each hand.
2. Bend at your knees and hips, keeping your back straight, your head up, and your eyes looking forward. Be sure to keep some of your weight back on your heels, keeping your knees from going forward past your toes. Lower your body to a position slightly higher than sitting in a chair.
3. As you slowly return to the starting position the resistance band should provide some resistance. Repeat ten to fifteen times.

# Front Rise

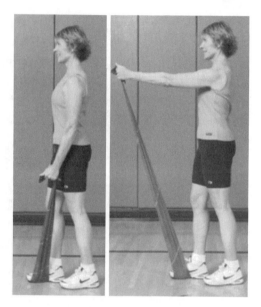

1. Start with the middle of the resistance band under one foot and one end in each hand. Stand with your feet shoulder-width apart and your knees slightly bent. Your hands should be in front of your thighs.
2. While maintaining a slight bend in your elbows, raise your arms until they are parallel with the floor.
3. Slowly lower your arms to the starting position and repeat ten to fifteen times.

# Pull-Down

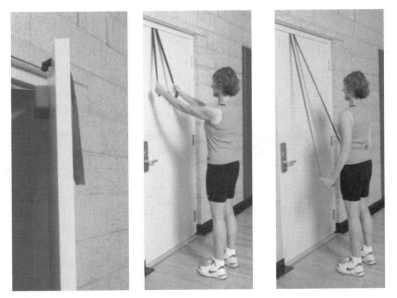

1. Tie a knot in the middle of a resistance band and close it securely in a door, allowing both ends to fall to the same side. They should be approximately the same length.
2. With your arms parallel to the floor, grip one end of the resistance band with each hand.
3. While maintaining a slight bend in your elbows, pull your arms down toward your thighs.
4. Slowly return to the starting position and repeat ten to fifteen times.

# Calf Exercise

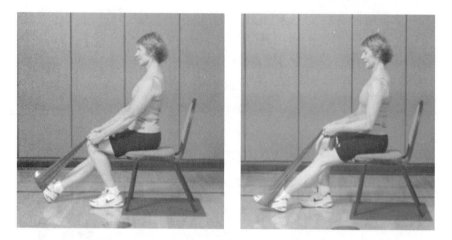

1. Sit upright in a chair or on a bench with one leg extended. Place the middle of the resistance band under that foot.
2. Using the band for resistance, point your toes. Maintain good posture throughout the exercise.
3. Slowly return to the starting position and repeat ten to fifteen times. Repeat on the opposite side.

# Bicep Curl

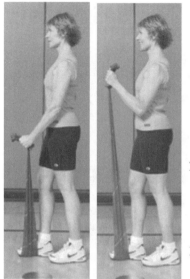

1. Stand with the middle of the resistance band under your feet and one end in each hand. Start with hands at your thighs with a slight bend in your elbows.
2. Bend your elbows, raising your hands up while your upper arms remain in a comfortable, fixed position at your sides.
3. Slowly return to the starting position and repeat ten to fifteen times.

# Tricep Extension

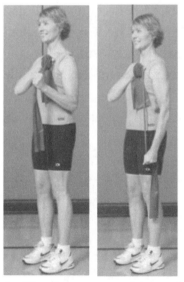

1. Stand with the resistance band in your right hand. Hold your right hand against the inside of your left shoulder where it should remain throughout the exercise. Allow most of the resistance band to hang free.
2. Grip the band six to eight inches below your right hand. Extend your left arm down to your side, keeping your upper arm in a comfortable, fixed position against your side.
3. Slowly return to the starting position and repeat ten to fifteen times. Repeat on the opposite side.

# Ball Squats

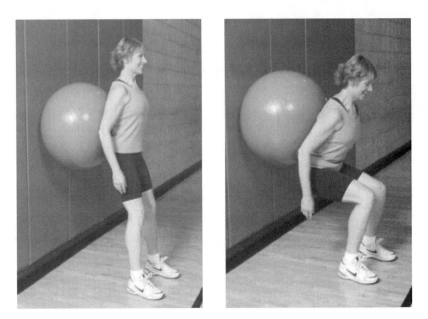

1. Begin by standing with the ball pressed between the wall and your lower back. Your feet should be in front of you about shoulder-width apart, with your knees slightly bent.
2. Slowly bend your knees, as if sitting down in a chair, while pushing your hips into the ball.
3. Slowly return to the starting position and repeat ten to fifteen times.

# Single-Leg Calf Rises

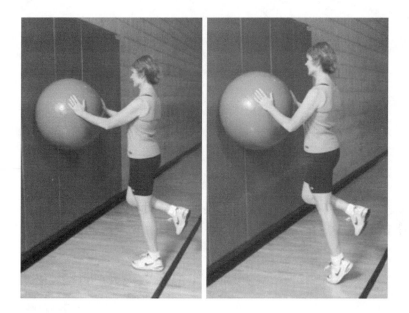

1. Stand on your left foot with the ball between your hands and the wall.
2. Raise straight up on your toes, lifting your heel off the floor. Do not lean into the ball.
3. Slowly lower to the starting position and repeat ten to fifteen times. Repeat on the other side.

# Ball Planks

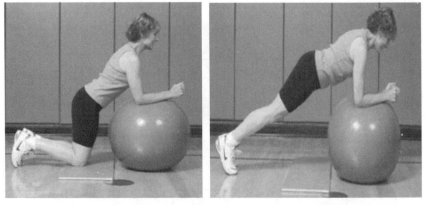

1. Start with your forearms on the ball and your knees on the floor.
2. Lift knees off the floor simultaneously, to a position in which your body is in a straight line.
3. Set a goal of holding this position for thirty to sixty seconds.

# Crunches

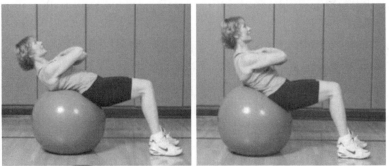

1. Sit on a ball and walk out until the ball is under your lower back. Your feet should be about shoulder-width apart.
2. Cross your arms across your chest.
3. Slowly curl up by raising your chest toward the ceiling, letting your shoulders and upper back lift off the ball.
4. Slowly return to the starting position. Set a goal of ten to twenty-five repetitions.

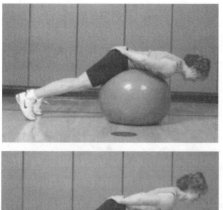

# Back Extension

1. Begin with the ball positioned under your stomach and both feet in contact with the floor. Rest your hands on the small of your back.
2. Slowly lift your chest slightly off the ball until the spine is straight or slightly extended.
3. Slowly return to the starting position. Set a goal of ten to twenty-five repetitions.

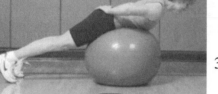

# Chest Press

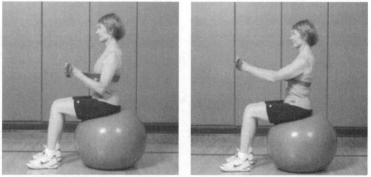

1. Sit upright on a ball, with a resistance band behind your back and under each arm. Place one end of the resistance band in each hand. Bend your elbows to about 90 degrees and keep your hands about chest height.
2. In a controlled motion, move your hands forward until your elbows are just slightly bent.
3. Slowly return to the starting position and repeat ten to fifteen times.

# Seated Row

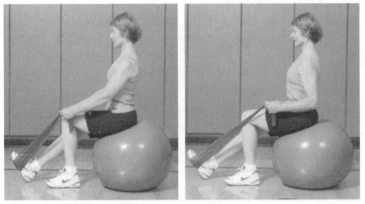

1. Sit on the ball with one leg extended. Wrap the middle of the resistance band under your foot and hold one end in each hand.
2. Start with your arms extended toward your foot. In a controlled motion, pull your elbows back while lifting your chest.
3. Slowly return to the starting position and repeat ten to fifteen times.

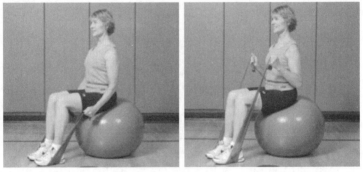

# Bicep Curl

1. Sit on the ball, with the middle of the resistance band under your feet and one end in each hand. Start with your hands at your thighs, with a slight bend in your elbows.
2. Bend your elbows, raising your hands while your upper arms remain in a comfortable, fixed position at your sides.
3. Slowly return to the starting position and repeat ten to fifteen times.

# Tricep Extension

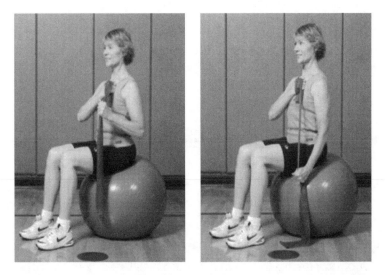

1. Sit on the ball, with the resistance band in your right hand. Hold your right hand against the inside of your left shoulder, where it should remain throughout the exercise. Allow most of the resistance band to hang free.
2. With your left hand grip the band six to eight inches below your right hand. Extend your left arm down to your side, keeping your upper arm in a comfortable, fixed position against your side.
3. Slowly return to the starting position and repeat ten to fifteen times. Repeat on the opposite side.

# Stretching Exercises

The exercises outlined in this basic stretching program are intended for individuals who are assumed to be healthy and not experiencing pain in the joints or back.

## BASIC STRETCHING GUIDELINES

With aging and a sedentary lifestyle, physiological changes occur to our musculoskeletal system and flexibility. Changes in joint flexibility can affect balance, mobility, and activities of daily living. By adding stretching exercises to your workout routine you can limit the reductions in flexibility that occur over time. It is important to warm up prior to stretching. Whether you are performing aerobic exercise, strength training, or both, be certain to begin and end your routine with five to ten minutes of light activity, followed by stretching.

## A FLEXIBILITY PROGRAM HAS THE FOLLOWING COMPONENTS:

- ♥ **Frequency:** Preferably stretching should be done most days.
- ♥ **Intensity:** Hold stretches until a *gentle* pull is felt in the muscle, not the joint. When the feeling of tension decreases, the stretch can be progressed.
- ♥ **Type:** Exercises in this section. Yoga, Tai Chi, Ai Chi, and Pilates are other examples.
- ♥ **Time:** Hold each stretch for fifteen to thirty seconds on both sides of your body.

♥ Progression: Try to gradually increase flexibility on stretches you find difficult but not painful. Do not try to gain too much range in one session. It may take weeks to see results.

## BASIC RULES OF POSTURE:

♥ Look straight ahead to keep the cervical spine properly aligned.
♥ If possible, your ears should be directly over your shoulders.
♥ Shoulders should be level and "squared," not slumped or rounded forward.
♥ A tall, elongated spine with your chest lifted, provides a strong position and decreases compression on the intervertebral discs.

## DO NOT STRETCH IF:

♥ A fracture is present
♥ The muscle or joint is inflamed (hot or swollen)
♥ You have been advised not to stretch a particular joint by a medical professional
♥ You are having pain with a particular stretch

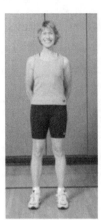
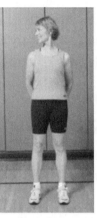

# Neck Stretch

1. Clasp hands behind your back.
2. Keep shoulders level.
3. Keeping your head level, rotate toward one side and hold.
4. Rotate toward the other side and hold.

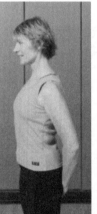
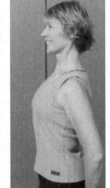

# Neck Stretch

1. Pull head straight back, keeping eyes and jaw level.
2. Do not allow your head to tilt up or down.

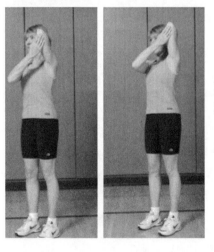

# Tricep Stretch

1. Raise the involved arm as if reaching overhead.
2. Drop hand behind your head.
3. If you already feel a stretch, hold that position.
4. If you are able, place opposite hand on elbow and gently press toward the back.

# Chest Stretch

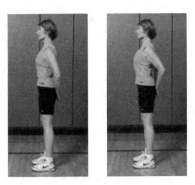

1. Clasp hands behind your back.
2. Roll shoulders back.
3. If necessary, slightly lift hands away from body without leaning forward.

# Chest Stretch

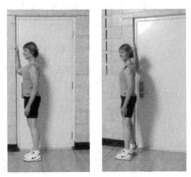

1. Place hand and elbow on a wall corner or doorframe at shoulder height.
2. Without moving the hand and elbow, take a step forward.
3. Turn entire body to face slightly away from the corner or doorframe.

# Quadricep Stretch (Standing)

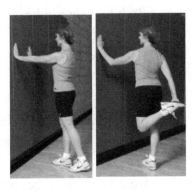

1. Hold onto a stable object for balance.
2. Lift the involved leg toward buttocks. Keep opposite knee slightly bent.
3. Grasp the ankle or pant leg with the opposite hand and gently pull.
4. Maintain an upright posture, keeping knees close together.

# Quadricep Stretch (Seated)

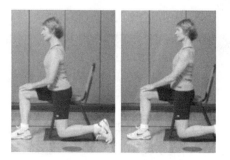

1. Using a chair, preferably without arm rests, move body to one side of the chair.
2. Lean trunk slightly forward and move involved leg back with your knee toward the floor.
3. Return trunk to upright position without moving leg.

# Calf Stretch

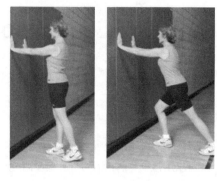

1. Place both hands against a wall and take a step back, slightly larger than a normal stride length.
2. Both feet should be pointed forward.
3. Keep the back leg straight and your heel on the ground.
4. Slowly move your weight forward, bending the front knee. Do not let your front knee move beyond your front foot.

# Achilles Stretch

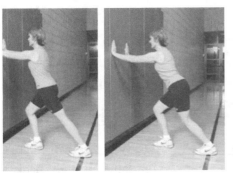

1. Take a step back, slightly larger than a normal stride length.
2. Both feet should be pointed forward.
3. Slowly move your weight forward, bending the front knee. Do not let your front knee move beyond your front foot.
4. Slightly bend your back knee keeping your heel on the floor.

# Hamstring Stretch (Seated)

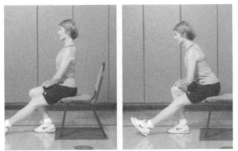

1. Position body near end of chair.
2. Keeping one leg bent at 90 degrees, extend opposite leg with heel resting on the floor.
3. Maintain a straight back and lean forward from the hips.
4. Keep chest and head lifted.

# Hamstring Stretch (Standing)

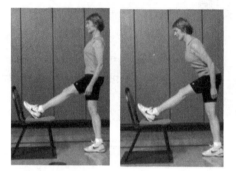

1. Place heel on the floor slightly in front of you, or on a low object.
2. Keeping the knee of the extended leg straight, slightly bend other knee.
3. Maintain a straight back and lean forward from the hips.
4. Keep chest and head lifted.

# NOTES

## CHAPTER 1

1. D. Levy, D. D. Savage, R. J. Garrison, K. M. Anderson, W. B. Kannel, and W. P. Castelli, "Echocardiographic Criteria for Left Ventricular Hypertrophy: The Framingham Heart Study," *American Journal of Cardiology* 59, no. 9 (April 15, 1987): 956–60; R. B. Devereux, E. M. Lutas, P. N. Casale, P. Kligfield, R. R. Eisenberg, I. W. Hammond, D. H. Miller, G. Reis, M. H. Alderman, and J. H. Laragh, "Standardization of M-Mode Echocardiographic Left Ventricular Anatomic Measurements," *Journal of the American College of Cardiology* 4, no. 6 (December 1984): 1222–30; D. W. Schwertz and P. M. Buttrick, "Gender Influences on Myocardial Structure and Function," in *Cardiovascular Health and Disease in Women*, 2nd ed., ed. Pamela S. Douglas (Philadelphia: W. B. Saunders, 2002).

## CHAPTER 3

1. W. C. Willett, A. Green, M. J. Stampfer, F. E. Speizer, G. A. Colditz, B. Rosner, R. R. Monson, W. Stason, and C. H. Hennekens, "Relative and Absolute Excess Risks of Coronary Heart Disease among Women Who Smoke Cigarettes," *New England Journal of Medicine* 317, no. 21 (November 19, 1987): 1303–309.

2. Ibid.; A. K. Sullivan, D. R. Holdright, C. A. Wright, J. L. Sparrow, D. Cunningham, and K. M. Fox, "Chest Pain in Women: Clinical, Investigative, and Prognostic Features," *British Medical Journal* 308, no. 6933 (April 2, 1994): 883–86.

3. J. W. Rich-Edwards, J. E. Manson, C. H. Hennekens, and J. E. Buring, "The Primary Prevention of Coronary Heart Disease in Women," *New England Journal of Medicine* 332, no. 26 (June 29, 1995): 1758–66.

4. American Heart Association, "Heart Disease and Stroke Statistics: 2007 Update at a Glance," http://www.americanheart.org/downloadable/heart/1166712318459HS_StatsInsideText.pdf [accessed November 24, 2007].

5. C. L. Ogden, M. D. Carroll, L. R. Curtin, M. A. McDowell, C. J. Tabak, and K. M. Flegal, "Prevalence of Overweight and Obesity in the United States, 1999–2004," *Journal of the American Medical Association* 295, no. 13 (April 5, 2006): 1549–55.

6. A. I. Qureshi, M. F. Suri, L. R. Guterman, and L. N. Hopkins, "Cocaine Use and the Likelihood of Nonfatal Myocardial Infarction and Stroke: Data from the Third National Health and Nutrition Examination Survey," *Circulation* 103, no. 4 (January 30, 2001): 502–506.

7. A. H. James, M. G. Jamison, M. S. Biswas, L. R. Brancazio, G. K. Swamy, and E. R. Myers, "Acute Myocardial Infarction in Pregnancy: A United States Population-Based Study," *Circulation* 113, no. 12 (March 28, 2006): 1564–71.

8. Ogden et al., "Prevalence of Overweight and Obesity," 1549–55.

9. American Heart Association, "Heart Disease and Stroke Statistics."

10. Ibid.

11. Ibid.

12. S. Booth-Kewley and H. S. Friedman, "Psychological Predictors of Heart Disease: A Quantitative Review," *Psychological Bulletin* 101, no. 3 (May 1987): 343–62.

# CHAPTER 4

1. American Heart Association, "Heart Disease and Stroke Statistics: 2007 Update at a Glance," http://www.americanheart.org/downloadable/heart/1166712318459HS_StatsInsideText.pdf [accessed November 24, 2007].

2. National Center for Health Statistics, "Health, United States, 2006," Centers for Disease Control and Prevention, http://www.cdc

.gov/nchs/hus.htm [accessed November 24, 2007].

3. J. M. Murabito, M. J. Pencina, B. H. Nam, R. B. D'Agostino Sr., T. J. Wang, D. Lloyd-Jones, P. W. Wilson, and C. J. O'Donnell, "Sibling Cardiovascular Disease as a Risk Factor for Cardiovascular Disease in Middle-Aged Adults," *Journal of the American Medical Association* 294, no. 24 (December 28, 2005): 3117–23.

4. G. Hu, P. Jousilahti, Q. Qiao, M. Peltonen, S. Katoh, and J. Tuomilehto, "The Gender-Specific Impact of Diabetes and Myocardial Infarction at Baseline and during Follow-Up on Mortality from All Causes and Coronary Heart Disease," *Journal of the American College of Cardiology* 45, no. 9 (May 3, 2005): 1413–18.

5. G. J. Blake, A. D. Pradhan, J. E. Manson, G. R. Williams, J. Buring, P. M. Ridker, and R. J. Glynn, "Hemoglobin A1c Level and Future Cardiovascular Events among Women," *Archives of Internal Medicine* 164, no. 7 (April 12, 2004): 757–61.

6. American Heart Association, "Heart Disease and Stroke Statistics."

7. W. C. Willett, A. Green, M. J. Stampfer, F. E. Speizer, G. A. Colditz, B. Rosner, R. R. Monson, W. Stason, and C. H. Hennekens, "Relative and Absolute Excess Risks of Coronary Heart Disease among Women Who Smoke Cigarettes," *New England Journal of Medicine* 317, no. 21 (November 19, 1987): 1303–309.

8. C. L. Ogden, M. D. Carroll, L. R. Curtin, M. A. McDowell, C. J. Tabak, and K. M. Flegal, "Prevalence of Overweight and Obesity in the United States, 1999–2004," *Journal of the American Medical Association* 295, no. 13 (April 5, 2006): 1549–55.

# CHAPTER 5

1. K. A. Bybee, T. Kara, A. Prasad, A. Lerman, G. W. Barsness, R. S. Wright, C. S. Rihal, "Systematic Review: Transient Left Ventricular Apical Ballooning: A Syndrome That Mimics ST-Segment Elevation Myocardial Infarction," *Annals of Internal Medicine* 141, no. 11 (December 7, 2004): 858–65.

2. L. Mosca, L. J. Appel, E. J. Benjamin, K. Berra, N. Chandra-Strobos, R. P. Fabunmi, D. Grady, C. K. Haan, S. N. Hayes, D. R. Judelson, N. L. Keenan, P. McBride, S. Oparil, P. Ouyang, M. C. Oz, M. E. Mendelsohn, R. C. Pasternak, V. W. Pinn, R. M. Robertson, K. Schenck-Gustafsson, C. A. Sila, S. C. Smith Jr., G. Sopko, A. L. Taylor, B. W. Walsh, N. K. Wenger, and C. L. Williams, "American Heart Association Evidence-Based Guidelines for Cardiovascular Disease Prevention in Women," *Circulation* 109, no. 5 (February 10, 2004): 672–93.

3. G. J. Balady, P. A. Ades, P. Comoss, M. Limacher, I. L. Pina, D. Southard, M. A. Williams, and T. Bazzarre, "Core Components of Cardiac Rehabilitation/Secondary Prevention Programs: A Statement for Healthcare Professionals from the American Heart Association and the American Association of Cardiovascular and Pulmonary Rehabilitation Writing Group," *Circulation* 102, no. 9 (August 29, 2000): 1069–73.

4. Ibid.

5. Ibid.

## CHAPTER 6

1. American Heart Association, "Heart Disease and Stroke Statistics: 2007 Update at a Glance," http://www.americanheart.org/downloadable/heart/1166712318459HS_StatsInsideText.pdf [accessed November 24, 2007].

2. Ibid.

3. Ibid.

4. T. L. Bush, E. Barrett-Connor, L. D. Cowan, M. H. Criqui, R. B. Wallace, C. M. Suchindran, H. A. Tyroler, and B. M. Rifkind, "Cardiovascular Mortality and Noncontraceptive Use of Estrogen in Women: Results from the Lipid Research Clinics Program Follow-up Study," *Circulation* 75, no. 6 (June 1987): 1102–109.

5. E. Barrett-Connor, M. A. Espeland, G. A. Greendale, J. Trabal, S. Johnson, C. Legault, D. Kritz-Silverstein, and P. Einhorn, "Postmenopausal Hormone Use Following a 3-Year Randomized Clinical

Trial," *Journal of Women's Health and Gender-Based Medicine* 9, no. 6 (July–August 2000): 633–43.

6. S. Hulley, D. Grady, T. Bush, C. Furberg, D. Herrington, B. Riggs, and E. Vittinghoff, "Randomized Trial of Estrogen Plus Progestin for Secondary Prevention of Coronary Heart Disease in Postmenopausal Women. Heart and Estrogen/Progestin Replacement Study (HERS) Research Group," *Journal of the American Medical Association* 280, no. 7 (August 19, 1998): 605–13; D. Grady, D. Herrington, V. Bittner, R. Blumenthal, M. Davidson, M. Hlatky, J. Hsia, S. Hulley, A. Herd, S. Khan, L. K. Newby, D. Waters, E. Vittinghoff, and N. Wenger (HERS Research Group), "Cardiovascular Disease Outcomes during 6.8 Years of Hormone Therapy: Heart and Estrogen/Progestin Replacement Study Follow-Up (HERS II)," Journal of the American Medical Association 288, no. 1 (July 3, 2002): 49–57.

7. J. E. Manson, J. Hsia, K. C. Johnson, J. E. Rossouw, A. R. Assaf, N. L. Lasser, M. Trevisan, H. R. Black, S. R. Heckbert, R. Detrano, O. L. Strickland, N. D. Wong, J. R. Crouse, E. Stein, and M. Cushman (Women's Health Initiative Investigators), "Estrogen Plus Progestin and the Risk of Coronary Heart Disease," *New England Journal of Medicine* 349, no. 6 (August 7, 2003): 523–34.

8. E. Barrett-Connor, D. Grady, A. Sashegyi, P. W. Anderson, D. A. Cox, K. Hoszowski, P. Rautaharju, and K. D. Harper (MORE Investigators), "Raloxifene and Cardiovascular Events in Osteoporotic Postmenopausal Women: Four-Year Results from the MORE (Multiple Outcomes of Raloxifene Evaluation) Randomized Trial," *Journal of the American Medical Association* 287, no. 7 (February 20, 2002): 847–57.

# CHAPTER 8

1. R. M. Krauss, R. H. Eckel, B. Howard, L. J. Appel, S. R. Daniels, R. J. Deckelbaum, J. W. Erdman Jr., P. Kris-Etherton, I. J. Goldberg, T. A. Kotchen, A. H. Lichtenstein, W. E. Mitch, R. Mullis, K. Robinson, J. Wylie-Rosett, S. St. Jeor, J. Suttie, D. L. Tribble, and T. L. Bazzarre,

"AHA Dietary Guidelines: Revision 2000: A Statement for Healthcare Professionals from the Nutrition Committee of the American Heart Association," *Circulation* 102, no. 18 (October 31, 2000): 2284–99.

2. L. W. Lissin and J. P. Cooke, "Phytoestrogens and Cardiovascular Health," *Journal of the American College of Cardiology* 35, no. 6 (May 2000): 1403–10.

3. C. D. Gardner, L. D. Lawson, E. Block, L. M. Chatterjee, A. Kiazand, R. R. Balise, and H. C. Kraemer, "Effect of Raw Garlic vs Commercial Garlic Supplements on Plasma Lipid Concentrations in Adults with Moderate Hypercholesterolemia: A Randomized Clinical Trial," *Archives of Internal Medicine* 167, no. 4 (February 26, 2007): 346–53.

4. M. H. Pittler and E. Ernst, "Ginkgo Biloba Extract for the Treatment of Intermittent Claudication: A Meta-Analysis of Randomized Trials," *American Journal of Medicine* 108, no. 4 (March 2000): 276–81.

5. L. Patrick and M. Uzick, "Cardiovascular Disease: C-Reactive Protein and the Inflammatory Disease Paradigm: HMG-CoA Reductase Inhibitors, Alpha-Tocopherol, Red Yeast Rice, and Olive Oil Polyphenols. A Review of the Literature," *Alternative Medicine Review* 6, no. 3 (June 2001): 248–71; D. Heber, I. Yip, J. M. Ashley, D. A. Elashoff, R. M. Elashoff, and V. L. Go, "Cholesterol-Lowering Effects of a Proprietary Chinese Red-Yeast-Rice Dietary Supplement," *American Journal of Clinical Nutrition* 69, no. 2 (February 1999): 231–36.

6. K. Linde, G. Ramirez, C. D. Mulrow, A. Pauls, W. Weidenhammer, and D. Melchart, "St John's Wort for Depression—An Overview and Meta-Analysis of Randomised Clinical Trials," *British Medical Journal* 313, no. 7052 (August 3, 1996): 253–58; R. C. Shelton, M. B. Keller, A. Gelenberg, D. L. Dunner, R. Hirschfeld, M. E. Thase, J. Russell, R. B. Lydiard, P. Crits-Cristoph, R. Gallop, L. Todd, D. Hellerstein, P. Goodnick, G. Keitner, S. M. Stahl, and U. Halbreich, "Effectiveness of St John's Wort in Major Depression: A Randomized Controlled Trial," *Journal of the American Medical Association* 285, no. 15 (April 18, 2001): 1978–86.

# CHAPTER 9

1. R. C. Ziegelstein, "Depression after Myocardial Infarction," *Cardiology in Review* 9, no. 1 (January–February 2001): 45–51.

2. S. Yusuf, S. Hawken, S. Ounpuu, T. Dans, A. Avezum, F. Lanas, M. McQueen, A. Budaj, P. Pais, J. Varigos, and L. Lisheng (INTERHEART Study Investigators), "Effect of Potentially Modifiable Risk Factors Associated with Myocardial Infarction in 52 Countries (The INTERHEART Study): Case-Control Study," *Lancet* 364, no. 9438 (September 11–17, 2004): 937–52.

# CHAPTER 10

1. W. B. Kannel and R. D. Abbott, "Incidence and Prognosis of Myocardial Infarction in Women: The Framingham Study," in *Coronary Heart Disease in Women*, ed. E. D. Eaker, B. Packard, and N. K. Wenger (Bethesda, MD: National Heart, Lung, and Blood Institute, National Institutes of Health, 1987); A. I. McGhie, M. Lim, and J. T. Willerson, "Nuclear Imaging," in *Heart Disease in Women*, ed. S. Wilansky and J. T. Willerson (New York: Churchill Livingstone, 2002), pp. 157–64.

2. M. J. Williams, T. H. Marwick, D. O'Gorman, and R. A. Foale, "Comparison of Exercise Echocardiography with an Exercise Score to Diagnose Coronary Artery Disease in Women," *American Journal of Cardiology* 74, no. 5 (September 1, 1994): 435–38.

3. E. Barasch, "Echocardiography," in *Heart Disease in Women*, ed. S. Wilansky and J. T. Willerson (New York: Churchill Livingstone, 2002), pp. 164–69.

4. D. Zhao, D. H. Freeman, and C. R. deFilippi, "A Meta-Analysis of Gender Differences in Exercise Testing," *Circulation* 94 (1995): I-497.

# CHAPTER 11

1. A. Carcagnì, M. Camellini, L. Maiello, M. Bocciarelli, G. Pastena, R. Bufalino, A. Morabito, E. Arbustini, and P. Presbitero, "Percutaneous Transluminal Coronary Revascularization in Women: Higher Risk of Dissection and Need for Stenting," *Italian Heart Journal* 1, no. 8 (August 2000): 536–41.

2. B. R. Brodie, "Why Is Mortality Rate after Percutaneous Transluminal Coronary Angioplasty Higher in Women?" *American Heart Journal* 137, no. 4, pt. 1 (April 1999): 582–84.

3. J. Mehilli, A. Kastrati, J. Dirschinger, H. Bollwein, F. J. Neumann, and A. Schömig, "Differences in Prognostic Factors and Outcomes between Women and Men Undergoing Coronary Artery Stenting," *Journal of the American Medical Association* 284, no. 14 (October 11, 2000): 1799–805.

4. D. Abramov, M. G. Tamariz, J. Y. Sever, G. T. Christakis, G. Bhatnagar, A. L. Heenan, B. S. Goldman, and S. E. Fremes, "The Influence of Gender on the Outcome of Coronary Artery Bypass Surgery," *Annals of Thoracic Surgery* 70, no. 3 (September 2000): 800–805; K. H. Humphries, M. Gao, A. Pu, S. Lichtenstein, and C. R. Thompson, "Significant Improvement in Short-Term Mortality in Women Undergoing Coronary Artery Bypass Surgery (1991 to 2004)," *Journal of the American College of Cardiology* 49, no. 14 (April 10, 2007): 1552–58.

5. E. Graves, "Detailed Diagnoses and Procedures, National Hospital Discharge Survey, 1987," *Vital and Health Statistics*, series 13, data from the National Health Survey, no. 100, DHHS Publication No. [PHS] 89-1761 (Washington, DC: US Government Printing Office, 1987); R. B. Devereux, "Valvular Heart Disease," in *Cardiovascular Health and Disease in Women*, 2nd ed., ed. P. S. Douglas (Philadelphia: W. B. Saunders, 2002).

# CHAPTER 12

1. "Genetic Disorders," in *Gene Therapy*, ed. J. Panno (New York: Facts on File, 2004), pp. 1–13.

2. We recommend Gregory Stock's *Redesigning Humans* for a thrilling introduction to the future prospects for genetic engineering.

# CHAPTER 13

1. Reported in the INTERHEART study. This discussion is adapted from an excellent article in *USA Today*, January 9, 2006. The primary scientific report appeared in *Lancet* 364, no. 9438 (September 11–17, 2004): 937–52.

2. H. O. Ventura, "Peripartum Cardiomyopathy: Clinical and Therapeutic Characteristics," *Journal of the Louisiana State Medical Society* 143, no. 5 (May 1991): 45–48; J. B. O'Connell, M. R. Costanzo-Nordin, R. Subramanian, J. A. Robinson, D. E. Wallis, P. J. Scanlon, and R. M. Gunnar, "Peripartum Cardiomyopathy: Clinical, Hemodynamic, Histologic and Prognostic Characteristics," *Journal of the American College of Cardiology* 8, no. 1 (July 1986): 52–56.

3. S. Brody and R. Preut, "Vaginal Intercourse Frequency and Heart Rate Variability," *Journal of Sex & Marital Therapy* 29, no. 5 (October–December 2003): 371–80.

4. M. Lameiras Fernández, M. González Lorenzo, and S. Alvarez Diéguez, "[Sexual Activity in Cardiac Patients: An Empirical Study]," *Atención Primaria* 26, no. 4 (September 2000): 249–54.

5. B. K. Johnson, "Sexuality and Heart Disease: Implications for Nursing," *Geriatric Nursing* 25, no. 4 (July–August 2004): 224–26.

6. R. DeBusk, Y. Drory, I. Goldstein, G. Jackson, S. Kaul, S. E. Kimmel, J. B. Kostis, R. A. Kloner, M. Lakin, C. M. Meston, M. Mittleman, J. E. Muller, H. Padma-Nathan, R. C. Rosen, R. A. Stein, and R. Zusman, "Management of Sexual Dysfunction in Patients with Cardio-

vascular Disease: Recommendations of The Princeton Consensus Panel," *American Journal of Cardiology* 86, no. 2 (July 2000): 175–81.

7. I. B. Addis, C. C. Ireland, E. Vittinghoff, F. Lin, C. A. Stuenkel, and S. Hulley, "Sexual Activity and Function in Postmenopausal Women with Heart Disease," *Obstetrics & Gynecology* 106, no. 1 (July 2005): 121–27.

8. C. Papadopoulos, P. Larrimore, S. Cardin, and S. I. Shelley, "Sexual Concerns and Needs of the Postcoronary Patient's Wife," *Archives of Internal Medicine* 140, no. 1 (January 1980): 38–41.

# GLOSSARY

**Aneurysm** A swelling of an artery, sometimes resembling the bulging of an old tube tire. *Aortic aneurysm* is a swelling, or enlargement, of the aorta—the main blood vessel of the body. Aneurysms are important because they can rupture.

**Angina** Pain in the chest caused by insufficient blood flow to the heart muscle. This pain is usually felt right behind the breastbone. It often produces a sensation of a crushing or pressurelike discomfort.

**Angina at rest** Chest pain that occurs without exertion or other provocation. This is a serious pattern of angina that requires prompt notification of your doctor.

**Angioplasty** The "plaque-busting" technique of inflating a balloon inside a coronary artery to relieve the narrowing. This is one of the techniques that can be done nonsurgically with a catheter in the catheterization laboratory.

**Antiarrhythmic** A drug used to combat an arrhythmia, or abnormal rhythm of the heart.

**Aorta** The large central artery that provides branches to supply blood to all organs of the body.

**Aortic dissection** A serious condition in which the wall of the aorta splits into two layers, creating a "double-barrel" aorta.

**Aortic valve** The main outflow valve of the heart. *Aortic stenosis* refers to narrowing of this valve. *Aortic regurgitation* refers to leaking of this valve.

**Arrhythmia** An abnormal rhythm of the heart.

**Arteriosclerosis** A thickening or hardening of artery walls due to a buildup of plaque or calcium, causing blockages and other cardio-vascular problems.

**Atrial septal defect** A small hole in the membrane that divides the two upper chambers or atria, of the heart. This has recently been implicated in causing migraine headaches.

**Atrium** The upper chamber of each side of the heart. There is a right and a left atrium. These chambers serve to preload, or boost, the action of the vital lower chambers, or ventricles, of the heart.

**Balloon pump** A small mechanical device placed into the aorta to assist the heart function. The balloon passes through the femoral artery in the leg to reach its position just behind the heart. The balloon is a temporary device. This device takes a great burden off the heart and can relieve otherwise resistant angina pains. This device can also be used to support a heart that is struggling after open heart surgery.

**Beta-blockers** An important and powerful class of drugs that decrease the rate and forcefulness of the heartbeat. These drugs are especially useful in the treatment of angina and arrhythmias.

**Block or heart block** A delay in the electrical impulses in the heart. There are three successive degrees of heart block, starting with a slight delay and progressing to irregular rhythms in which there is a danger that the heart will stop completely.

**Bradycardia** A slow heart rate, defined as one below sixty beats per minute. This can cause dizziness or loss of consciousness.

**"Broken heart" syndrome** A phenomenon in which a woman can experience the symptoms of a heart attack related to an emotional event or trauma, but without any corresponding physiological causes. Doctors still aren't certain why this condition is triggered in some women under great emotional or mental stress, but with medical treatment most affected women make a full recovery.

**Calcium channel blockers** An important and powerful class of drugs that dilate the arteries of the heart, helping to get more blood to the heart muscle. They also dilate the arteries of the body, lowering blood pressure and relieving the workload of the heart. These drugs can furthermore decrease the heart rate, helping to treat arrhythmias.

**Cardiomyopathy** Weakening of the heart muscle. The term comes from the Greek "cardia," or *heart*, and "pathia," or *weakness*. Cardiomyopathy is called *ischemic* if it results from heart attacks or *idiopathic* if it is of unknown cause.

**Catheterization** An essential type of cardiac test in which wires and tiny tubes are passed into the heart to permit measurement of pressures in the heart, visualization of the strength and contraction pattern of the heart, and detailed assessment of the coronary arteries for possible blockages. This is the "gold standard" of cardiac diagnostic tests.

**Congestive heart failure** A state of excess fluid in the lungs and legs, due to backup of water behind weak pumping chambers of the heart. There are many possible causes of this problem.

**Coronary artery** One of the small arteries that run on the surface of the heart and provide nourishment to the heart muscle. It is the coronary arteries that become blocked and cause heart attacks.

**Coumadin** A powerful blood thinning medication. Another name for this drug is Warfarin. It is used for patients with mechanical heart valves or with atrial fibrillation.

**Defibrillator** The paddle device used to convert dangerous heart rhythms to normal ones by powerful electrical discharge.

**Diastole** The passive filling phase of the cardiac cycle, in which the powerful ventricles wait passively, preparing for the active contraction to come.

**Echocardiogram or "echo"** A test using sound waves, like sonar, to obtain images of your heart. This test can disclose problems with the valves of your heart or with the pumping strength of your heart. It is a comfortable and easy test to take. At times, your doctor may order or perform a transesophageal echocardiogram, in which the echo probe is passed through your throat into the esophagus, or swallowing tube. This type of echo gives superb images of your heart, as the probe lies just behind the heart inside your body.

**Edema** The medical term for swelling from water retention. This is usually manifested in the ankles. It can be a sign of heart failure, as well as other physical problems. The edema may show an imprint if you press your thumb against the swollen skin.

**Ejection fraction** A measure of the pumping strength of the left ventricle, the most important pumping chamber of the heart. This value represents the proportion of blood ejected with each heartbeat. A normal value is 70 percent. If the ejection fraction falls below 40 percent, then symptoms of inadequate pumping strength of the heart may appear.

**Electrocardiogram or EKG** An electrocardiogram, or test of the electrical signals of your heart. This is a simple and easy test, which can show evidence of inadequate blood flow to the heart, heart attack, or abnormal rhythm of the heart.

**Electrophysiologic (or EP) test** A test for patients with a history of or who may be at risk for severe cardiac arrhythmia. The test is done by tickling the heart electrically via a catheter passed into the chambers of the heart.

**Embolus** (also embolism) A traveling particle in the bloodstream. This is often a particle of arteriosclerotic debris or clot. In the systemic circulation, this may be devastating if the particle travels to the heart (coronary arteries) or to the brain. On the pulmonary side of the circulation, these particles may go to the lung (pulmonary embolism), causing difficulty breathing or even shock and death.

**Endocarditis** Infection of a heart valve, which is a type of bloodstream infection. This is a serious problem that can destroy the valve tissue. Antibiotics and/or surgery are always required.

**Fibrillation** A fast, chaotic heart rhythm. Ventricular fibrillation, affecting the powerful lower heart chambers, is a very serious rhythm disturbance that invariably causes cardiac arrest. Atrial fibrillation, affecting the upper chambers of the heart, is more common and much more benign.

**Heart-lung machine** The mechanical device that takes over the functions of the heart and the lungs while the most intricate segments of open heart surgery are performed. It includes a pump to circulate the blood and an artificial lung. The heart-lung machine is colloquially called, in professional circles, simply, "the pump."

**Heart murmur** An abnormal sound heard through a stethoscope, representing turbulent flow across a dysfunctional heart valve. A murmur may be present because of either narrowing or leaking of the affected valve.

**Heparin** A powerful blood thinner, usually given intravenously, especially for blood clots, heart attacks, or artificial heart valves. This drug is especially useful because it wears off within two to four hours, unlike oral blood thinners, which can take days to dissipate.

**Holter monitor** A continuous tape recording of your EKG done by a portable machine while you go about your daily life. This is used to look for arrhythmias—abnormal heart rhythms—which may not be detected on a "spot" EKG while you are in the doctor's office.

**Hormone therapy (HT)** A prescribed treatment of estrogen, usually with progestin, a synthetic form of progesterone. This treatment compensates for the loss of sex hormones that occurs with menopause. It should be used only for the short-term relief of symptoms of menopause and is not appropriate for the prevention of chronic diseases such as osteoporosis and heart disease. Estrogen therapy alone is only recommended for women who have had their uterus removed, as it can cause uterine cancer in women who do not use it with progestin.

**Hypertension** High blood pressure. This is defined as a pressure exceeding 140/90 millimeters of mercury.

**Hypertrophy** A state in which the main pumping chamber of the heart—the left ventricle—becomes thick and muscle-bound from pressure overload. This is a harmful condition.

**Inflammation** The medical term for irritation of tissues. This irritation may be from infection or from noninfectious causes. Many authorities feel that inflammation is an important cause of arteriosclerosis and coronary artery disease.

**Internal mammary artery** The artery that runs inside the chest wall just beside the breastbone. It gets its name because it normally supplies blood to the breast. We "borrow" this artery for use in supplying blood to the heart. This artery is the most durable conduit for the coronary artery bypass operation.

**Mitral valve** The main inflow valve of the heart. Mitral stenosis refers to narrowing of this valve. Mitral regurgitation refers to leaking of this valve.

**Myocardial infarction** The technical term for a heart attack, or death of a portion of the heart muscle. This is usually caused by blockage of one of the coronary arteries, which supply blood and oxygen to the heart muscle.

**Pericardiectomy** Surgical removal of the pericardial sac, necessary in cases of severe pericardial disease.

**Pericardium** The thin, glistening, flexible but inelastic (non-stretchable) sac that surrounds the heart in its central position in the chest. Replacement heart valves are fashioned from the pericardia of cows.

**Plaque** A thick material composed of cholesterol fats, circulating cells from the bloodstream, and tissue cells that attach to artery walls and can cause a buildup leading to possible cardiac problems. It can also rupture into the bloodstream, causing blood clots and possible heart attacks. Angioplasty is the procedure in which the plaque is busted away, usually by a method of balloon dilation.

**Prolapse** Excess backward movement of a heart valve leaflet. Usually applied to the mitral valve. Mitral valve prolapse can often be a completely benign, or mild, condition.

**Pulmonary edema** A state of flooding of the lungs with fluid backed up behind a weak heart. Shortness of breath is usually profound. This is a very serious manifestation of congestive heart failure.

**Regurgitation** Backward leakage through a heart valve.

**Restenosis** A long-term repeat narrowing of a site in the arteries following the surgical insertion of a stent. Drug-eluting stents are used to help prevent this from happening.

**Rheumatic fever** An infection, usually occurring during childhood or early adulthood, which can affect the heart and heart valves. Problems with valve function may occur years later, in adult life. Rheumatic fever may follow untreated sore throats, caused by the streptococcus bacterium.

**Sinus node** The spot of tissue in the right atrium that initiates an electrical signal to trigger heartbeats. A problem in the sinus node could cause fainting (syncope) or arrhythmias. A pacemaker is sometimes needed to replace the function of the sinus node.

**Stenosis** A narrowing, as in an artery or a cardiac valve.

**Stent** The fine metal "fencing" often used to supplement an angioplasty procedure. The stent stays permanently inside the stretched artery, serving to keep the blockage from pushing its way again into the open channel of the artery.

**Stress test** A test in which a stress is placed on your heart, either by having you exercise or by giving you a powerful medication. This test is used to screen for blocked coronary arteries or to assess the impact of known blockages. During this test, the doctor will check to see if you are feeling chest pain, if your EKG changes, or if images taken by nuclear or echo means show any abnormalities. The exercise for this test is usually performed on a treadmill, thus many doctors refer to this as the "treadmill test."

**Syncope** The medical term for fainting.

**Systole** The active phase of cardiac contraction, during which the powerful ventricles eject blood from the heart.

**Tachycardia** A very rapid heart rate. This could be the sign of a dangerous underlying cardiac disease if caused in the ventricles, the lower chambers of the heart.

**Thrill** A vibration felt by the examiner's hand placed over the heart in cases with very loud heart murmurs. The presence of a thrill represents intensely turbulent flow across a very abnormal heart valve.

**Thrombosis** Blood clots (thrombus) form in the veins or arteries, which can lead to heart attacks or strokes. This is sometimes caused when patients with stented arteries stop taking anti-platelet drugs. When clots occur in the legs and are transported to the lungs, it is called deep vein thrombosis (or DVT).

**Transmural myocardial infarction** A heart attack that goes all the way through the heart wall. This is more extensive and more serious than a nontransmural heart attack.

**Unstable angina** Angina of increasing pattern, occurring more frequently, lasting longer, requiring more nitro pills for control, or even occurring without exertion or other provocation. Unstable angina may presage a heart attack and should be promptly reported.

**Ventricle** The lower pumping chamber of each side of the heart. There is a right and a left ventricle. These are the important pumping chambers of the heart.

# INDEX

Illustrations are indicated by *italicized* page numbers.

low-density lipoprotein. *See* LDL cholesterol
lungs, 31
  pulmonary edema, 151. *See also* edema
  pulmonary embolus, 45. *See also* embolus
  pulmonary hypertension, 34
  *See also* heart-lung machine
Lyme disease, 62

ma huang, 133
mammary artery, 167
  left vs. right used in bypass grafts, 177–78
Marfan's syndrome, 35, 211
mechanical valves, 36, *185*, 186–88
median sternotomy, 190
medications, 36, 70
  antirejection drugs, 199, 202
  drug-eluting stents, 162–63
  effectiveness of herbal and natural supplements, 131–37
  SERMs, 118
  used in hormone therapy, 106
  used to treat heart disease, 123–29
  used to treat osteoporosis, 118
  *See also* ACE inhibitors; angiotensin II receptor blockers; antiarrhythmic medications; aspirin; beta blockers; blood, blood thinning medications; calcium channel blockers; diuretics; fibrates; lipid-altering medications; *names of specific prescription drugs*; *specific heart problems*; statins
Menest, 106
menopause, 74, 77, 103–105
  and heart disease, 107–108
  myth that only postmenopausal women are at risk for heart disease, 13, 14, 16–17
  perimenopause, 74, 104
  premenopause, 74, 79, 85, 104, 106, 223
  symptoms, 105
  women protected from arteriosclerosis until, 223–25
  *See also* hormone therapy (HT)
meolazone, 124
metabolic syndrome, 139–40
metolazone, 124
metoprolol, 124
Mevacor, 126
Micronized (natural progesterone) pill, 106
micturition syncope, 64
migraines, 226–27
minimally invasive or noninvasive surgery, 66–67, 161
  minimal incision in mitral valve surgery, 229
  *See also* angioplasty
mini-Maze, 66
ministrokes, 120